T0214461

Pediatric Tricky Topics, Volume 2

Christine M. Houser

Pediatric Tricky Topics, ·Volume 2

A Practically Painless Review

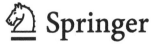 Springer

Christine M. Houser
Department of Emergency Medicine
Erasmus Medical Center
Rotterdam, The Netherlands

•

ISBN 978-1-4939-3108-8   ISBN 978-1-4939-3109-5   (eBook)
DOI 10.1007/978-1-4939-3109-5

Library of Congress Control Number: 2014949915

Springer New York Heidelberg Dordrecht London

Printed on acid-free paper

Springer Science+Business Media LLC New York is part of Springer Science+Business Media (www.springer.com)

To my parents, Martin and Cathy, who made this journey possible, to Patrick who travels it with me, and to my wonderful children Tristan, Skyler, Isabelle, Castiel, and Sunderland who have patiently waited during its writing – and are also the most special of all possible reminders of why pediatric medicine is so important.

Important Notice

Medical knowledge and the accepted standards of care change frequently. Conflicts are also found regularly in the information provided by various recognized sources in the medical field. Every effort has been made to ensure that the information contained in this publication is as up to date and accurate as possible. However, the parties involved in the publication of this book and its component parts, including the author, the content reviewers, and the publisher, do not guarantee that the information provided is in every case complete, accurate, or representative of the entire body of knowledge for a topic. We recommend that all readers review the current academic medical literature for any decisions regarding patient care.

Preface

Keeping all of the relevant information at your fingertips in a field as broad as pediatrics is both an important task and quite a lot to manage. Add to that the busy schedule most physicians and physicians-to-be carry of a practice or medical studies, family life, and sundry other personal and professional obligations, and it can be daunting. Whether you would like to keep your knowledge base up to date for your practice, are preparing for the general pediatric board examination or recertification, or are just doing your best to be well prepared for a ward rotation, *Pediatric Tricky Topics*, *Volume 2*: *A Practically Painless Review* can be an invaluable asset.

This book brings together the information from several major pediatric board review study guides, and more review conferences than any one physician would ever have time to personally attend, for you to review at your own pace. It's important, especially if there isn't a lot of uninterrupted study time available, to find materials that make the study process as efficient and flexible as possible. What makes this book additionally unusual among medical study guides is its design using "bite-sized" chunks of information that can be quickly read and processed. Most information is presented in a question-and-answer format that improves attention and focus, and ultimately learning. Critically important for most in medicine, it also enhances the speed with which the information can be learned.

Because the majority of information is in question-and-answer (Q & A) format, it is also much easier to use the information in a few minutes of downtime at the hospital or office. You don't need to get deeply into the material to understand what you are reading. Each question and answer is brief – not paragraphs long as is often the case in medical review books – which means that the material can be moved through rapidly, keeping the focus on the most critical information.

At the same time, the items have been written to ensure that they contain the necessary information. Very often, information provided in review books raises as many questions as it answers. This interferes with the study process, because the learner either has to look up the additional information (time loss and hassle) or skip the information entirely – which means not really understanding and learning it. This book keeps answers self-contained, meaning that any needed information is provided either directly in the answer or immediately following it – all without lengthy text.

To provide additional study options, questions and answers are arranged in a simple two-column design, making it possible to easily cover one side and quiz yourself, or use the book for quizzing in pairs or study groups.

For a few especially challenging topics, or for the occasional topic that is better presented in a regular text style, a text section has been provided. These sections precede the larger Q & A section for that topic (so, for example, allergy & immunology text sections precede the question-and-answer section for allergy & immunology). It is important to note that when text sections are present, they are not intended as an overview or introduction to the Q & A section, although some may provide useful preparatory material for that section. They are intended to be stand-alone topics simply found presented as clearly written and relatively brief text sections.

The materials utilized in *Practically Painless Pediatrics* have been tested by residents and attendings preparing for the general pediatric board examination, or the recertification examination, to ensure that both the approach and content are on target. All content has also been reviewed by attending and specialist pediatricians to ensure its quality and understandability.

If you are using these materials to prepare for an exam, this can be a great opportunity to thoroughly review the many areas involved in pediatric practice, and to consolidate and refresh the knowledge developed through the years so far. *Practically Painless Pediatrics* books are available to cover the breadth of the topics included in the General Pediatric Board Examination.

The formats and style in which materials are presented in *Practically Painless Pediatrics* utilize the knowledge gained about learning and memory processes over many years of research into cognitive processing. All of us involved in the process of creating it sincerely hope that you will find the study process a bit less onerous with this format, and that it becomes – at least at times – an exciting adventure to refresh or build your knowledge.

Brief Guidance Regarding Use of the Book

Items which appear in **bold** indicate topics known to be frequent board examination content. On occasion, an item's content is known to be very specific to previous board questions. In that case, the item will have "popular exam item" or "item of interest" beneath it.

Some topics cross over between different subjects; for example retinopathy of prematurity is relevant to both the *Practically Painless Pediatric* neonatology book and the ophthalmology section of this book. In that case, items on the topic will be present in both books, although more extensive coverage of certain aspects will be found in one versus the other. To preserve completeness of coverage, some items for those topics will be found in each of the sections; however complete repetition of the items in multiple sections would render the chapters unnecessarily long. It is therefore important to review both sections to ensure a full coverage of the relevant material, if the purpose is preparation for the pediatric board exam or recertification.

At times, you will encounter a Q & A item that covers the same content as a previous item within the same chapter. These items are worded differently, and often require you to process the information in a somewhat different way, compared to the previous version. This variation in the way questions from particularly challenging or important content areas are asked is not an error or oversight. It is simply a way to easily and automatically practice the information again. These occasionally repeated items are designed to increase the probability that the reader will be able to retrieve the information when it is needed – regardless of how the vignette is presented on the exam, or how the patient presents in a clinical setting.

Occasionally, a brand name for a medication or piece of medical equipment is included in the materials. These are indicated with the trademark symbol (®) and are not meant to indicate an endorsement of, or recommendation to use, that brand name product. Brand names are sometimes included only to make processing of the study items easier, in cases in which the brand name is significantly more recognizable to most physicians than the generic name would be.

The specific word choice used in the text may at times seem informal to the reader, and occasionally a bit irreverent. Please rest assured that no disrespect is intended to anyone or any discipline, in any case. The mnemonics or comments provided are only intended to make the material more memorable. The informal wording is often easier to process than the rather complex or unusual wording many of us in the medical field have become accustomed to. That is why rather straightforward wording is sometimes used, even though it may at first seem unsophisticated.

Similarly, visual space is provided on the page, so that the material is not closely crowded together. This improves the ease of using the material for self- or group quizzing, and minimizes time potentially wasted identifying which answers belong to which questions.

The reader is encouraged to use the extra space surrounding items to make notes or add comments for himself or herself. Further, the Q & A format is particularly well suited to marking difficult or important items for later review & quizzing. If you are utilizing the book for exam preparation, please consider making a system in advance to indicate which items you'd like to return to, which items have already been repeatedly reviewed, and which items do not require further review. This not only makes the study process more efficient & less frustrating, but it can also offer a handy way to know which items are most important for last-minute review – frequently a very difficult "triage" task as the examination time approaches.

Finally, consider switching back and forth between topics under review, to improve processing of new items. Trying to learn & remember many information items on similar topics is often more difficult than breaking the information into chunks by periodically switching to a different topic.

Ultimately, the most important aspect of learning the material needed for board and ward examinations is what we as physicians can bring to our patients – and the amazing gift that patients entrust to us in letting us take an active part in their health.

With that focus in mind, the task at hand is not substantially different from what each examination candidate has already done successfully in medical school & in patient care. Keeping that uppermost in our minds, board examination studying should be both a bit less anxiety provoking and a bit more palatable. Seize the opportunity and happy studying to all!

Rotterdam, The Netherlands   Christine M. Houser

About the Author

Christine M. Houser completed her medical degree at the Johns Hopkins University School of Medicine, after spending 4 years in graduate training and research in Cognitive Neuropsychology at George Washington University and the National Institutes of Health (NIH). Her Master of Philosophy degree work focused on the processes involved in learning and memory, and during this time she was a four-time recipient of training awards from the NIH. Dr. Houser's dual interests in cognition and medicine led her naturally toward teaching, and "translational cognitive science" – finding ways to apply the many years of cognitive research findings about learning and memory to how physicians and physicians-in-training might more easily learn and recall the vast quantities of information required for medical studies and practice.

Content Reviewers

Many thanks to Dr. Robert Yetman, Professor and Director of the Residency Program in the Division of Community and General Pediatrics at the University of Texas – Houston Medical School in Houston, Texas, for his tireless assistance in reviewing the manuscript, and coordinating its content review.

For Allergy and Immunology Topics

Joyce Hsu, MD
Instructor in Allergy and Immunology
Brigham & Women's Hospital
Harvard Medical School
Boston, MA, USA

Anand Gourishankar, MD
Assistant Professor of Pediatrics
University of Texas – Houston Medical School
Houston, TX, USA

For Hematology and Oncology Topics

Adam L. Green, MD
Attending in Pediatric Hematology-Oncology,
Boston Children's Hospital/Dana-Farber Cancer Institute
Instructor of Pediatrics, Harvard Medical School
Boston, MA, USA

For Nephrology Topics

Craig B. Woda, MD, PhD
Nephrology Fellow
Department of Pediatrics
Harvard Medical School
Boston Children's Hospital
Boston, MA, USA

Heather C. Moore, MD
Assistant Professor of Pediatrics
University of Texas – Houston Medical School
Houston, TX, USA

For Urology Topics

Mark D. Hormann, MD
Assistant Professor of Pediatrics
University of Texas – Houston Medical School
Houston, TX, USA

For Dermatology Topics

Ines Wu Soukoulis, MD
Instructor in Dermatology
Harvard Medical School
Boston Children's Hospital
Boston, MA, USA

Misti Ellsworth, DO
Assistant Professor of Pediatrics
University of Texas – Houston Medical School
Houston, TX, USA

Sutapa Khatua, MD
Assistant Professor of Pediatrics
University of Texas – Houston Medical School
Houston, TX, USA

For Ophthalmology Topics

Miriam Ehrenberg, MD
Department of Ophthalmology
Schneider Children's Medical Center of Israel
Petach Tikvah, Israel

Mfon Ekong, MD
Assistant Professor of Pediatrics
University of Texas – Houston Medical School
Houston, TX, USA

For Ear, Nose, and Throat Topics

Amalia Guardiola, MD
Assistant Professor of Pediatrics
University of Texas – Houston Medical School
Houston, TX, USA

For Adolescent Medicine and Relevant Gynecology Topics

Monaliza Evangelista, MD
Assistant Professor of Pediatrics
University of Texas – Houston Medical School
Houston, TX, USA

Contents

Chapter 1
Selected Allergy and Immunology Topics

Immunology Basic Topics

Some aspects of the immune system are ready to defend us all the time – without any special experience or priming from other parts of the immune system. These aspects of the immune response are called "innate immunity." Examples of the innate immune system are the skin and mucosal barriers of the body, and cells such as macrophages, neutrophils, natural killers, and the complement system.

These systems do not develop a "memory" for antigens they have seen in the past, and their response to the antigen will not improve with experience.

"Acute-phase reactants" are part of the innate immunity system. When the macrophages encounter something that might be dangerous, they send out TNF, IL-1, and IL-6. This stimulates the liver to synthesize the acute-phase reactant proteins. Some acute-phase reactants can actually bind to bacteria, activating the complement system to kill the bacteria.

Immune processes that require prior experience with an antigen, or special priming of the cell to get its functions started, are called "adaptive" or "acquired immunity." This type of immunity is possible only with experience with the environment, so it is acquired, rather than innate. For example, when a B-cell is primed to function by interactions with an activated helper T-cell, that is an example of acquired immunity. When a specific antibody is made to match an antigen encountered in the body, the immune system is "adapting" its response according to what it encounters – hence the term "adaptive" immunity.

Macrophages actually function as part of both the innate and adaptive immune system. If they encounter something that looks foreign to them, they eat it up – acting as an innate defense mechanism. Additionally, though, they present fragments of what they ate on their cell surface, in an MHC-II complex. This presentation serves to activate both B- and T-cells, making the macrophage a critical initiator of the adaptive immune response, along with other antigen-presenting cells.

© Springer Science+Business Media New York 2016
C.M. Houser, *Pediatric Tricky Topics, Volume 2*,
DOI 10.1007/978-1-4939-3109-5_1

B-cells can also present antigens to T-cells, in MHC-II complexes on their surfaces. Polymorphonuclear leukocytes (PMNs), on the other hand, cannot present antigen, even though they seem similar to macrophages in terms of their eating habits.

The B-cell receptor (BCR) for binding antigens is incredibly skilled – it can be designed to recognize virtually any type of molecule. T-cells only see short peptides (in MHC-II complexes).

Major Histocompatibility Types

Generally speaking, MHC-II is found on cells of the immune system, and is used for presentation of antigen. MHC-I is usually found on nonimmune system body cells. It is used to recognize self, but can also display foreign antigens, in some cases (e.g., viral infection of a cell).

Immune Systems for Identifying & Destroying Threats

The Complement System

The goal of the complement system is to poke holes in foreign invaders that don't belong in the body. Complement "fixing" means that complement complex has been attached to a cell's surface, or to an antibody-antigen complex on the cell, and the cell is likely to now be lysed. The complement system is part of innate immunity.

There are three pathways of complement system activation. All of them culminate in formation of a *membrane attack complex (MAC)*.

The *classic pathway* (it was the first discovered – nothing really classic about it!) of complement fixation occurs when an antigen-antibody (Ag-Ab) complex gets the interest of complement factor C1. It attaches to the cell associated with the Ag-Ab complex.

After a series of conversions, C5b+C6+C7 insert themselves into the cell membrane.

When C8 and C9 join them they are called *the MAC*. The MAC opens a hole in the cell's membrane, lysing it. (A "MAC attack" – kind of like what you see at McDonalds®!)

The *alternative pathway* doesn't require any help from antibodies. It is part of the innate immune system, and relies on the ready supply of complement factor C3b in the body. (Some C3 is spontaneously converted to C3b at a baseline level in the body. It is this C3b that is used in the alternative pathway.) Some bacteria, fungi, and clumps of IgA stimulate this complement to "fix" on their target without any other molecules being present.

The alternative pathway *begins with complement factor C3b* (the opsonin), and then involves factors *B, D, and properdin*. It ends, as always, with a MAC attack (C5b+C6+C7, joined by C8 & C9).

The third pathway is called the *lectin pathway*, because it is activated when polysaccharides present on pathogens bind to lectin or ficolin molecules of the body's innate immune system. The lectin pathway successfully targets certain bacterial, viral, and fungal pathogens, including the RSV virus and *Neisseria* strains of bacteria.

The Story of Antibody-Mediated (Humoral) Immunity –

1. A macrophage presents a bit of antigen in its MHC-II complex, on the cell's surface.
2. A helper T-cell binds to the macrophage, recognizing the antigen in the MHC-II complex.

    a. The helper T-cell starts to make:

        i. IL-2   T-cell growth factor
       ii. IL-4   B-cell growth factor
      iii. IL-5   B-cell differentiation factor
       iv. IL-6   B-cell activation/IgG production factor

3. The matching B-cell is also activated by binding with the macrophage MHC-II complex containing the antigen, and through direct binding with the T-cell through surface receptors (CD40 & CD40L).
4. Stimulation from IL-4 and other molecules leads the B-cell to activate into a plasma cell (immunoglobulin-secreting cell), and divide to provide many daughter cells, or to become a memory cell.

"T-cell-independent antigens" are antigens that stimulate B-cells directly, without any assistance from the T-helper cells.

The Story of Cell-Mediated Immunity –

Type IV Hypersensitivity

1. A macrophage and a bacterium meet. The macrophage eats the bacteria, and throws some pieces of it into an MHC-II on its own surface.
2. The matching CD4+ T-helper cell wanders by, and binds with the macrophage MHC-II complex holding the antigen. The T-cell is "activated" by this process, and starts to proliferate. T-cell proliferation generates a "clone" of the same antigen-specific T-helper cell. T-cell activation and proliferation mainly occur when the T-cell is stimulated with IL-1 (from the macrophages) and IL-2 (from lymphocytes).
3. The excited macrophages, together with the excited and proliferating T-helper cells, then produce a Type 4 delayed hypersensitivity reaction.

Cytotoxic Destruction

1. A virus invades a cell in the gut.
2. Viral envelope glycoproteins turn up on the invaded cell's surface, presented in MHC-I complexes.
3. A matching CD8+ cytotoxic T-cell wanders by, and realizes that the MHC-I cup contains its matching antigen. This stimulates it to divide into a clonal line of cells. (IL-2 from involved CD4+ helper T-cells is important in this process.)
4. The clones of the cytotoxic T-cell go out to find cells with the right MHC-I and antigen pairing. When they find them, they secrete perforins to open the cells' membranes and kill the infected cells.

Types of Cells Involved in the Immune Response

T-cells

T-cells carry "CD" surface markers. All T-cells are marked with CD2 and CD3. They proliferate, in general, when they encounter IL-2.

The helper cells (both Th1 and Th2) are marked with CD4 and CD28 molecules on their surface. They activate when their CD28 receptor binds the B7 surface marker on antigen-presenting cells. They are stimulated to divide and produce a clone line by IL-2.

Cytotoxic T-cells are CD8+. They are also stimulated by IL-2.

Regulatory T-cells are a subset of T-cells that moderate immune activation and maintain self-tolerance. (Previously, these cells were termed suppressor T-cells, but that was not an accurate reflection of what they do, so they were renamed.)

About 70 % of the body's T-cells are helper cells. About 75 % of the circulating lymphocytes are T-cells (rather than B-cells, or other lymphocyte types).

Memory T-cells are formed, in addition to memory B-cells. (However memory B-cells get most of the attention, due to their impressive IgG response, when activated.)

T-cells mature in the thymus, and are selected for further development based on the response they have to self molecules. Those that react against self are deleted (die). The process is called "clonal deletion" and is also referred to as "negative selection."

T-cells are also *positively selected*. This means that the T-cell must be able to interact with MHC proteins from the self. If they can't, they won't be able to facilitate the immune response, so they are also killed.

Natural Killer or NK cells

These are large, granular, white cells that do not develop in the thymus. They also do not carry the T-cell surface markers (neither CD4 nor CD8), although they are part of the "lymphocyte family tree."

NK cells kill tumor cells and virally infected cells without ever having antigen presented to them. Actually, they target cells that do not have MHC-I surface markers, or have fewer markers than normal. Often, the body's cells lose their MHC-I markers when they are infected or malignant.

B-cells

B-cells are critical to the production of antibody. They carry markers on their surface for B7, and the antigen they are looking for (IgM or IgD molecules specific to the antigen, embedded on their surface, called B-cell receptors, or BCR). They are stimulated to divide and produce antibody by IL4 and IL5.

Macrophages

Come from "myeloid" precursors, so they are not in the same family tree as lymphocytes or granulocytes (eosinophils, basophils, and neutrophils). They eat, and present antigen. They do not have antigen-recognizing receptors on their surface. They also make up the "reticuloendothelial" or "mononuclear phagocyte system," part of the immune system, which refers to macrophage-like cells parked in the various tissues, and especially in liver, and spleen. In the liver, they are Kupffer cells.

Macrophages are activated by gamma-interferon. They also secrete many cytokines that stimulate various cells, including liver production of acute-phase reactants like C-reactive protein.

Functions of Immune System Cells

B-cells – The main functions of the B-cells are to provide defense against bacterial invasion, through antibodies. (Additionally, antibodies can sometimes bind to toxins, inactivating them. Sometimes, antibodies can bind to viruses, and inactivate them, as well.)

B-cells are also involved in allergy, such as hay fever, because they contribute the IgE (Type I hypersensitivity). They are also involved in various other autoimmune processes, mainly due to their production of antibody.

T-cells – The main functions of T-cells are to defend against viruses and fungus. T-cells also have an important role against *Mycobacterium tuberculosis*, and are the main cells responsible for the reaction in the TB skin test (an example of a Type IV delayed hypersensitivity reaction, all of which are T-cell mediated). They also monitor for tumor cells, and destroy them when they see them.

T-cells are also important in certain allergies, such as poison oak and poison ivy.

T-helper cells are crucial for the regulation of the B-cell antibody response.

T-cells are very important in graft rejection.

Lab Tests That Use the Immune System

Tests of Agglutination
(How much something sticks to something else)

In general, agglutination tests check whether a particular antibody and antigen are present in a sample. Depending on the particular test, you could be checking for the presence of antibody, or antigen. The tests the blood bank runs to identify different blood types and groups fall into this category.

For example, if the blood bank wants to know whether a patient's blood has the blood type B markers (both B and AB would have the marker), they combine samples of the patient's blood with a sample of marker B antibodies. If they agglutinate, the blood is either type B or AB. If it does not, the blood type is either A or O.

There are two special tests of agglutination you need to have a working knowledge of, the direct and indirect Coombs tests. The Coombs test is mainly used to evaluate whether there is an immune reason for a hemolytic anemia.

Direct Coombs Test

This version of the Coombs checks whether the RBCs already have antibody coating their surface. If so, an immune reaction against the RBCs was in full swing, whether the patient's own immune system was doing it or the mother's immune system was attacking the fetal blood.

The test is simple. Antibodies against human IgG are added to the blood sample you're interested in. If these antibodies agglutinate the blood, the sample was already coated in antibody. (The anti-IgG antibody sticks to the Fc part of the antibodies already on the cell's surface. It "cross-links" different cells together, because the two Fab-binding sites can bind to IgG on two different cell bodies. This makes them stick together.)

Indirect Coombs Test

In this version of the test, there is an extra step. That is what makes it "indirect." You evaluate serum you think *might* be able to attack RBCs. No attack has happened yet.

The patient's serum is added to laboratory RBCs with the marker of interest (for example, blood type B). The "serum" part of the blood contains whatever antibodies the patient has circulating in the bloodstream. Then you add the anti-human IgG antibodies just as you did for the direct test. If antibodies for the marker were present, then the cells will agglutinate when they are combined with both the serum and the anti-human IgG.

The indirect test is typically used to check for Rh incompatibilities, so that the physician will know whether an Rh-negative mother has been sensitized to Rh-positive cells. (When performing the test, the blood cells should otherwise match Mom's, so you know your results depended on the Rh factor.) Mom's serum is combined with known Rh+ cells. Anti-human IgG is added. If Mom's serum contains antibodies that coat the RBCs, then the anti-human IgG will agglutinate them. If Mom does not have antibodies to Rh+ cells, then antibody should not be on the cells, and no agglutination should occur.

Direct and indirect fluorescent antibody tests are exactly the same idea as direct and indirect Coombs tests. It's just that in this case, another batch of antibodies is added as a final step. If these antibodies find their match, a positive result is detected by fluorescence, rather than agglutination.

Tests of Precipitation

These tests look for soluble antigen or soluble antibody. If enough of either is present, combining the two results in precipitation, because the antigen-antibody complexes cross-link and "fall out" of solution, due to being too complex or heavy.

The *radial immunodiffusion test* is a traditional type of precipitation test. This test can be used to measure the amount of the different types of immunoglobulins present in a patient's serum. It is done on an agar plate, with a known amount of antibody to each of the different immunoglobulin types added to a particular spot in the agar. The diameter of the precipitation allows you to conclude approximately how much of each immunoglobulin type is present in that patient's serum. This test can be used to measure the approximate quantity of any substance for which an antibody is available, not only immunoglobulins.

Radioimmunoassays & ELISA

These tests can be used if you need to evaluate lower levels of antigen or antibody, than in the tests above. They are more sensitive than the agglutination- or precipitation-based tests.

Antigen is coated onto plates, and serum is added, followed by addition of labeled antibody recognizing human immunoglobulin. Areas with human antibody bound to its antigen can then be identified.

The ELISA is, of course, very important because it is the initial screening test for HIV. It has many false positives however. Due to the relatively high false-positive rate (appropriate for a screening test), a positive result should always be confirmed with a follow-up Western blot test.

ELISA testing is now able to provide both qualitative information (whether the antigen-antibody complex is present) and the quantity or concentration of the target item. ELISAs are in use for detection of toxins and confirmation of pathogen presence (e.g., *E. coli* enterotoxin and mycobacteria in tuberculosis).

Western Blot

This specific protein detection test is important as a confirmatory test for HIV infection. Viral antigens (or other antigens, depending on what is being tested) are separated by gel electrophoresis, and transferred (blotted) onto a special type of membrane. Patient serum is then added. If HIV-specific antibodies are present, they will bind to the antigens stuck on the membrane, in different areas, representing clumps of particular antigens.

Finally, specially labeled anti-human IgG antibodies are added. They "stick to" any antigen-bound antibodies from the test serum. A sort of developer is added that causes a color to appear on the membrane where anti-human IgG is bound. The pattern and intensity of spots can then be interpreted to indicate which circulating antibodies were present in the serum. In the case of HIV testing, if the correct pattern of colored spots appears, it indicates that the patient has antibodies against the proteins of the HIV virus, confirming that he or she has been exposed to the virus.

Hypersensitivity Reactions

Type 1 – Immediate Hypersensitivity Reactions (start within minutes)

Local Atopy
  Anaphylactic Shock (whole-body response)
  Requires previous sensitization/exposure, and is caused by IgE.
  Cross-linking of antigens to IgE antibodies already sitting on the surface of the mast cell or basophil causes them to dump their inflammatory granules. If cells in the skin do this, it produces a local reaction. Basophils will do this in the circulation, increasing the likelihood of systemic response.
  Histamine release creates the typical "wheal and flare" hive pattern on the skin.
  Some types of asthma (in response to environmental allergens), as well as allergic rhinitis (hay fever), fall into this category. Foods are a common trigger for anaphylaxis in children.
  Anaphylactoid shock, now more commonly known as pseudoanaphylaxis, refers to a patient presentation that looks like anaphylaxis, but that was actually not caused by IgE mechanisms in the immune system.

Type 2 – Cytotoxic Hypersensitivity Reactions (Start hours to about a day after exposure.)

Antibody-dependent cell-mediated cytotoxicity – but *not* IgE.
  Previous sensitization or exposure *not* needed.
  Usually known as cytotoxic hypersensitivity, damage occurs when antibodies direct the immune system to attack cells that are performing a useful function in the body. These are usually "self" cells, but can also be "borrowed" cells, such as those from a blood transfusion. The antibodies involved are generally IgM or IgG.
  The antibodies may target actual self structures (intrinsically or innately part of the individual), or in some cases, they target a foreign protein that has attached itself

to a part of a self cell. For example, some infections or drug exposures may cause foreign molecules to be attached to otherwise healthy cells or body surfaces.

Once the antibodies have targeted the cells or tissues, cytotoxic destruction follows. Cells are destroyed through various immune mechanisms, including activation of the classical complement pathway, and direct cytotoxic destruction from natural killer cells and macrophages.

Examples are Goodpasture's syndrome, drug-induced hemolytic anemia, transfusion reactions, and hemolytic disease of the newborn.

Type 3 – Immune Complex Reactions (Start about 1 week after exposure, typically, but varies from hours to multiple weeks.)

Immune complex (antigen bound to antibody) damage.

Previous sensitization not required.

Small circulating antigen-antibody complexes are deposited in various body tissues. This stimulates the immune system to attack those tissues, because they seem to be "marked for destruction" by the antibody attached to an antigen.

Complement induces an inflammatory response. Neutrophils and macrophages will invade the area and damage necessary body cells, while mast cells degranulate, adding to inflammation. (Chemotactic factors are produced to draw neutrophils and macrophages to the area, through complement mechanisms.)

Complement, clotting factors, phagocytes, and anaphylatoxin (from the complement pathway) promote damage to the tissue harboring the immune complex.

Examples include: Serum sickness (foreign serum injected into someone producing immune complexes)
Polyarteritis nodosa – Ag-Ab complexes deposit in arteriolar walls
Arthus reaction – rare reaction requiring prior sensitization
Thrombus, hemorrhage, and necrosis occur in the skin due to severe inflammatory response
Rheumatoid arthritis

Type 4 – Delayed-Type Hypersensitivity Reactions (Cell Mediated) (Start 2 to 3 days after exposure)

Cell mediated *only!* No antibodies involved.

Previous sensitization not required (it develops during the exposure, over time).

This reaction involves T-cells that require time for activation and expansion, hence its name.

Macrophages present antigens on their surface that are recognized by T-helper cells. The macrophages get overexcited by cytokines coming from the T-cell system. The two cell types stimulate each other, driving a cycle of local inflammation and tissue damage. They tend to collect in areas around vessels. Granulomas can sometimes form, if the antigen remains in the area long enough. Activated CD8+ T cells are also involved, directly killing cells in the area.

Example: Contact dermatitis, and reaction to TB test (*very commonly used example*), Type 1 diabetes mellitus

Transplant Issues & Immunology

Possible types of tissue grafts

Allografts – As with other related "allo" words, allografts refer to transplanting materials between two nonidentical members of the same species. Most of our usual transplant scenarios involve this type of transplant. (For example, transplanting a kidney from one individual to another.)

Isograft – Transplant between genetically identical twins, or sometimes between very genetically similar research animals. Another word for this is "syngeneic" (syn – same, geneic – genes).

Autograft – Transplanting something from one site to another on the same individual (for example, using leg veins for cardiac bypass surgery).

Xenograft – Transplanting across species – does not work well!

What is graft vs. host disease?

This is a very specific situation that can occur when donor tissue that is, itself, still immunocompetent is put into a host who is not.

T-cells are the main culprits in graft vs. host disease.

The main problem is that the outside T-cells (the ones from the donor that were contained in the graft) see that the host is not what they were expecting. They recognize the host as foreign, by looking at the MHC molecules. They attack the host's cells, in a *type IV hypersensitivity reaction*. Antibodies are not involved in graft vs. host disease.

How will the patient present in graft vs. host disease?

Patients usually present with skin rash, diarrhea, and jaundice (dermatitis, enteritis, & hepatitis). Treatment consists of immunosuppression. When graft vs. host disease develops >100 days after onset, it is even more serious, and includes obstructive pulmonary disease, neurologically mediated weakness, pain, and muscle cramps, along with weight loss.

Rejection reactions – Not the same as graft vs. host!

There are several types of rejection reactions, and the different reactions are mediated by different parts of the immune system. Rejection is the host attacking the organ – that is how it is different from graft vs. host disease.

Hyperacute rejection –
Hyperacute rejection is what it sounds like – it happens really quickly. Rejection of the foreign organ happens in minutes to hours, so the graft never "takes."

How could rejection occur so quickly? Just as with any immune response, if it happens very quickly then it must depend on either innate immune mechanisms, such as complement, or preformed antibodies. Although the host has not seen the donor organ before, in some cases he or she does have antibodies to the tissue, based on prior exposures to transfusions, fetuses, etc. Complement is also active in the acute rejection process.

Why is hyperacute rejection also known as "white graft reaction?" Because the organ almost immediately turns white, after initially turning pink when the vessels were connected and blood flow restored. The white color results from the rapid vessel constriction and occlusion that occurs with this severe immune response.

Accelerated rejection –
Accelerated rejection occurs over a few days. Reactivation of previously sensitized T-cells gets this type of rejection response going.

This type of rejection is also called a "second set" reaction, because it usually occurs when a second transplant from the same individual is given to a donor after their body rejected the first transplant!

Accelerated rejection is actually an "acute rejection" of the transplant. Acute rejection is described next. Accelerated rejection is acute rejection that happens faster than usual.

Acute rejection –
Acute rejection takes days to weeks to develop. It takes longer because it is a primary activation of T-cells against the foreign antigens on the new organ.

T-helper cells activate cytotoxic T-cells via IL-2 to go kill cells in the graft or organ.

T-helper cells activate macrophages via interferon-gamma to go eat the cells. TNF release by the macrophages encourages more lymphocytes to invade the area.

In acute rejection, the organ swells, and the site may be tender. In kidney transplantation, in particular, acute rejection harms the transplanted kidney because it damages the renal vessels.

Chronic rejection –
Develops over months or years. There are often many episodes of rejection, separated by periods of quiescence. Antibodies and immune complexes are part of the process, but cell-mediated toxicity is also involved.

With repeated episodes, fibrosis and vascular occlusion occur and increase. Organ function is eventually lost due to the repeated episodes of organ damage.

MHC Matching

Matching the major histocompatibility complexes is one of the great challenges facing our current transplant techniques. MHC genes in humans are called human leukocyte antigens (HLA). Molecules that are synthesized under the direction of the HLA genes vary tremendously, and the HLA genes received from father and mother are expressed codominantly in the child – that is why it is so difficult to find organ donor matches among unrelated individuals.

HLA genes are coded on chromosome 6. Each individual has two haplotypes of HLA molecules, as mentioned above, one from the mother and the other from the father. If both haplotypes can be matched between the donor and recipient, the probability of successful transplant is higher (about 95 % for kidneys at 5 years) than it is if only one haplotype can be matched (about 80 % for kidneys at 5 years).

Possible donor and recipient pairs are matched for their HLA types, by comparing the relevant DNA sequences. Donor and recipient should also be compatible, of course, for Rh and ABO blood types.

To evaluate whether a donor and recipient are HLA matches, two of the important laboratory tests are the mixed lymphocyte assay, and the microcytotoxicity assay.

Mixed Lymphocyte Assay

The mixed lymphocyte assay evaluates how well the two sets of B and T cells can get along. T-cells from the host and B-cells from the donor are incubated together. The B-cells are actually only present to stimulate the T-cells, and the B-cells are irradiated in advance to ensure that they won't proliferate and confuse the results of the assay.

If the T-cells "notice" the MHC differences on the new cells, they proliferate. If they don't, they just sit around.

A positive result on the mixed lymphocyte assay is expressed in terms of the amount of thymidine the cells take up. That is because the cells are using the thymidine for DNA synthesis. The amount of thymidine they take up, then, is an indirect measure of how much they have divided.

Because this test involves the B- and T-cells, it is targeting whether the MHC-II markers are compatible or not.

Microcytotoxicity Assay

The microcytotoxicity assay, on the other hand, targets MHC-I compatibility. Antisera known to be toxic to certain MHC-I antigens is mixed with the donor cells and complement. If the antibodies in the antisera recognize the MHC-I as foreign, they will bind, complement will be activated, and the cell will lyse.

A positive result on the microcytotoxicity assay is entry of dye into the cell (meaning that its membrane is now open to the dye, courtesy of the complement MAC complex).

Immuno Trivia

Which cell in the human body lacks MHC markers? Red blood cells – cells without nuclei do not normally carry MHC markers.

Chapter 2
General Allergy and Immunology Question and Answer Items

Which MHC class of molecules are present on the immune cells of the body?

MHC-II

Which body cells have no MHC markers?

Red blood cells

Which group of immune cells cannot "see" an antigen *at all*, unless it is sitting in an MHC-II molecule?

T cells – CD4+ type

How is an "HLA" related to the "MHC?"

Consider them the same – Technically, HLA is for humans

Which lymphocytes can attack things even if the targets have neither MHC-I nor MHC-II molecules on their surface?

Natural killer (NK) cells

What is the main function of CD4+ T-helper cells?

To stimulate antibody production by B-cells (& B cell maturation)

How do CD4+ T-helper cells get activated?

By encountering MHC-II molecules loaded with antigen on other immune system cells (antigen-presenting cells)

© Springer Science+Business Media New York 2016
C.M. Houser, *Pediatric Tricky Topics, Volume 2*,
DOI 10.1007/978-1-4939-3109-5_2

There are actually two types of CD4+ T-cells – the helpers (which increase B cell antibody production) and what other group?

Regulatory CD4+ T cells (previously known as suppressor-inducer cells)

What does a regulatory T cell do?

Suppresses immune activation. They are important in regulating the development of autoimmunity

The overall impact of CD4+ T-cells on antibody production (by B cells) is _____?

Regulation (up or down, depending on which CD4+ cells are active)

If a cell is CD56+ and CD16+, what kind of T cell is it?

Natural killer

There are two populations of CD8+ T cells. What are they?

1. Cytotoxic
2. Regulatory
(modifying B cell antibody production)

Which class of T cells is most important in defending against viruses and cancer?

Cytotoxic CD8+

What two important classes of surface markers are on the surface of B cells?

Immunoglobulins

&

MHC-II

What two events stimulate B cells to become plasma cells?

Interacting with CD4+ cells

Or

Direct interaction with antigen

Which type of immunoglobulin is found in various body secretions?

IgA

Which type of immunoglobulin is secreted when the immune system begins its response to a new antigen?

IgM

What is special about the structure of IgM?

It's huge
(Five immunoglobulins joined like a big snowflake – officially called a "pentamer")

Which immunoglobulin is the *main* one, in the body's antibody response?

IgG

Which antibody is secreted when the body sees an antigen it has fought in the past?

IgG

If the initial immune system response is to produce IgM, and the later response is IgG, how does that happen?

"Class switching"

(The B cell changes from IgM production to IgG production)

IgM is usually found as a pentamer. IgA, on the other hand, is usually found as what type of structure?

As a dimer (2 IgAs joined together)
+
a secretory piece
(the secretory piece is added by the epithelial cells, during processing for secretion)

How is the structure of IgA different, when it is in the serum?

It is a monomer

What are the two areas of an immunoglobulin molecule called? (created in the lab by partially digesting the protein)

Fab
&
Fc

There are also two regions of immunoglobulin molecules, which correspond to the two sections of the immunoglobulin. What are they?

The constant region
&
variable "antibody-binding" region

(the variable region is made up of both the light chain & part of the heavy chain)

Which part of the immunoglobulin is variable, with a huge number of possible shapes to bind antigen?	Fab region (As in Fab fragments to bind things up) (Ab = antigen-binding region)
Which part of the immunoglobulin activates complement, or sometimes other immune cells, to eliminate bound antigens?	Fc region (c = cell or complement-binding area) *C also equals constant region*
Which type of immunoglobulin has four different subtypes?	IgG
Which type of immunoglobulin *both* crosses the placenta and is also found in breast milk?	IgG (IgA is also in breast milk, but it doesn't cross the placenta)
Which portion of the immune system is referred to as the "humoral" system?	The B cell portion
Which portion of the immune system is called the "cellular" immune system?	The T cell portion (even though plenty of other cells are also involved)
SCID refers to "severe combined immune deficiency." Which sets of immune cells are often deficient in this "combined" disorder?	B & T cells *(sometimes also NK cells – various combinations are possible within the diagnosis "SCID")*
Why is SCID often missed in the neonatal period?	Lymphocyte counts are "abnormally" high during infancy, so their lymphocyte count may appear normal, and neonates are often not exposed to life-threatening infections that would reveal the faulty immune system
Why are more infants within the USA now being diagnosed with SCID very early?	Since 2008, a variety of states have added SCID to their newborn screening program (with good success in detecting SCID infants)
What is the lower limit for absolute lymphocyte count at birth?	$2,500/mm^3$

Which infectious etiologies are SCID children at increased risk for?

<u>All</u> of them

By what age would you expect SCID patients to present, and how do they typically present?

By 3 months –
Typically with recurrent or persistent thrush, diarrhea, respiratory infections, & failure to thrive

What anatomic abnormality is classically seen on the chest X-ray of an infant with SCID?

No visible thymus
(missing "sail sign")

What vaccinations should you not give to patients with SCID?

No live attenuated vaccines!

What is the most common way to inherit SCID?

X-linked
(47 % of US cases)

If SCID is not inherited as an X-linked disorder, it is usually inherited in what fashion?

Autosomal recessive
(variety of mechanisms)

(most common in Europe)

What is special about transfusing an SCID patient?

Blood must be irradiated to destroy the foreign WBCs

(leukocyte depletion is NOT sufficient)

If a SCID patient receives a blood transfusion that has not been irradiated, what is the problem?

The foreign T cells may initiate a graft-versus-host disease *against the patient*

The second most common cause of SCID, after X-linked, is what specific cause?

Autosomal recessive purine salvage problems
(about 20 %)

Which two enzyme problems lead to purine salvage SCID?

Adenosine deaminase (ADA)
(15 % of cases)

&

Purine nucleoside phosphorylase (PNP)
(around 4 % of cases)

While we often hear about ADA deficiency as a cause of SCID, we don't often hear about PNP. Why not?	It is less common & Less severe
What other body system is often abnormal in SCID patients whose underlying problem is ADA deficiency?	Skeleton (especially pelvic dysplasia & costochondral joint abnormalities) Mnemonic: Think of a skeletal gal named "ADA" who "scids" and injures her axial skeleton!

How do SCID patients with PNP deficiency (purine nucleoside phosphorylase) present differently from ADA deficiency patients?
    (3 ways it's better)
    (2 ways it's worse)
	• Presents later
	• Less severe
	• No skeletal issues
	
	• + Neurological problems
	• + Autoimmune problems

How is SCID usually treated?	**Bone marrow transplant** (supportive care, until BMT is arranged)
For ADA-deficiency SCID patients, what temporary treatment is available, until bone marrow transplant can be arranged?	Bovine ADA enzyme replacement
If your patient has normal platelets and RBCs, *but almost no white cells*, what is the diagnosis?	SCID – due to "reticular dysgenesis"
Reticular dysgenesis SCID is fatal in infancy unless what treatment is completed?	Bone marrow transplant
The treatment of choice for all forms of SCID is _____?	Bone marrow transplant
Which two unusual causes of pneumonia are common in SCID children?	PCP (due to *P. jiroveci*) & viral interstitial pneumonia (due to adenovirus, CMV, etc.)

Regardless of the underlying problem, SCID patients should all have what lab finding?

Low absolute lymphocyte count

In reticular dysgenesis, the lymphocytes & granulocytes are both missing. Which cell populations are normal?

Platelets & RBCs

If a vignette states that your patient is missing B & T cells, *yet the number of natural killer cells (another type of lymphocyte) is normal*, what gene is mutated?

RAG 1 or 2
(known as RAG 1 or 2 deficiency)

SCID resulting from mutations in RAG1 and RAG2 would lead to which lymphocyte populations being absent?

T cells and B cells

(due to inability to repair double-stranded breaks formed during rearrangement)

Partial inactivation of the RAG 1 or 2 genes results in what syndrome?

Omenn

Mnemonic: Think of it as "omit" syndrome –
part of the gene has been "omitted"

Omenn syndrome develops when genes important to what special immune cell process are altered?

The V (D) J rearrangement genes

(these genes are important to the big diversity of antibodies the immune system can form, and also the diversity of antigen-type receptors found on B & T cells)

Immune deficiency + skin problems, diarrhea, & hepatosplenomegaly = what SCID-related syndrome?

Omenn syndrome

Omenn syndrome consists of lymphopenia & what three major symptoms/signs?

1. Skin problems (especially exfoliative erythroderma)
2. Diarrhea
3. HSM

Some children are born without MHC-II molecules. What is the name for their disorder?

MHC class II deficiency syndrome

(sensible enough name!)

Patients with MHC class II deficiency are especially likely to get which kinds of infections?

Viral!

They are have significant risk for pyogenic bacterial infections and opportunistic infections, but much less than is seen in SCID

What is the ultimate treatment for MHC class II deficiency?

Bone marrow transplant is the treatment of choice – but it may or may not fully cure the disorder

Non-hematopoietic cells are still missing the MHC II marker, which can impair important cell-to-cell interactions

If a patient's SCID disorder is not an X-linked disorder, it is very likely to be what type of inheritance pattern?

Autosomal recessive

(Example: ADA deficiency)

If a pediatric patient has chronically high IgM levels, he or she will likely have low levels of what other immunoglobulins?

IgG, IgA, IgE

(all immunoglobulin types that require class switching)

How is hyper-IgM syndrome inherited?

X-linked (more common)

&

Autosomal recessive (very rarely)

Which has the better prognosis, X-linked or autosomal recessive hyper-IgM syndrome, and why?

- Autosomal recessive
- Second decade risk of malignancy much higher for X-linked (especially liver cancer)

What is the underlying problem with hyper-IgM syndrome?

CD40 molecules are defective. CD40 is needed for Ig class switching (e.g., IgM → IgG)

If a patient has a defect in CD40 or CD40L, what immunodeficiency will this cause?

Hyper-IgM syndrome – a type of immunodeficiency

(due to inability of T cells to activate B cells)

What are hyper-IgM patients given to reduce the chance of infection occurring?

IVIG
(& TMP/SMX for PCP prophylaxis)

Why are hyper-IgM patients routinely given trimethoprim-sulfamethoxazole?

High risk for PCP (also known as *Pneumocystis jiroveci*)

How is hyper-IgM syndrome treated?

Trick question – it depends:
- **X-linked – bone marrow transplant**
- **Recessive – IVIG & TMP/SMX**

Boys with X-linked hyper-IgM syndrome often have what type of related disorders?

Autoimmune

Do you expect any abnormalities on physical exam of a patient with hyper-IgM syndrome?

Hepatosplenomegaly

&

Enlarged lymph nodes

An infant boy presents with *recurrent otitis media* in the *first year of life*. His older brother is having difficulty with OM and frequent sinus infections. He has *large lymph nodes*, and HSM. What test should you send?

Immunoglobulin studies

What is "common variable" immuno-deficiency?

A (heterogeneous) group of immune disorders with:

Low-level production of most Ig types & difficulty making specific antibodies

B cell numbers are sometimes alright in common variable immunodeficiency, so what is the problem with the Ig?

The B cells don't turn into plasma cells very well (so not much Ig is made)

(T cell abnormalities are also involved for many patients, but their role in the disorder is not fully understood)

Can common variable immunodeficiency patients have a normal total IgG?

Yes – sometimes (but still immunocompromised)

If the serum IgG level is sometimes normal, why are common variable patients at increased risk of infection?	High-quality antibodies specific to a particular antigen cannot be made in quantity
How is common variable immunodeficiency different from SCID? (2 points)	• B cells are present, they just don't differentiate well • T cells are present
Common variable immunodeficiency (CVID) patients have frequent infections in what three parts of the body, especially?	• Lungs • Gut • Sinuses
What gut problem often accompanies common variable immunodeficiency?	Sprue-like malabsorption (and diarrhea) *(Also due to Giardia!)*
When nodules are biopsied in CVID patients, what is a common finding?	Non-caseating granuloma
In addition to a sprue-like illness, are common variable patients likely to have other autoimmune-type problems?	Yes – Anemias & arthritides
How are common variable immunodeficiency patients managed, in terms of infection?	IVIG & antibiotics (as needed)
Are males or females more often affected by common variable immunodeficiency?	Affects both genders equally (multiple genetic mechanisms)
DiGeorge syndrome has a variety of immune system manifestations. It usually results from deletion of which chromosome area?	**22q11**

In addition to immune abnormalities, what else is expected in DiGeorge syndrome?
(4 items)

Heart problems
Facial abnormalities
Hypoparathyroidism
Intellectual disability

Low calcium + immune abnormalities in an infant or young child = (consider) what diagnosis?

DiGeorge syndrome

What does "complete" DiGeorge syndrome refer to?

Complete absence of the thymus & parathyroid glands –
T cells are absent
B cells are normal

Just 1 % of DiGeorge syndrome patients have this form . . .

If normal B cells are present, but there are no T cells, what are the consequences (if any) for B cell function?

B cells generally will not produce much antibody without T cell stimulation (except in the special case of "thymic-independent antigens")

"Complete" DiGeorge syndrome will present identically to what other disorder?

SCID –
Despite the normal *number* of B cells

If complete DiGeorge syndrome patients are clinically the same as SCID patients, then what must you worry about with transfusions of blood?

Graft-versus-host disease
(transfusions must be irradiated)

What treatment is available for complete DiGeorge syndrome patients?
(3 options)

Thymic transplant

Bone marrow transplant
(results unclear to date)

&

IVIG

Immunologically speaking, how do "partial" DiGeorge children present?

- **Normal B cell function**
- **Partial T cell deficiency**

What is the usual course of partial DiGeorge syndrome?

Improves over time
(reason not clear)

Which is more common, complete or partial DiGeorge?

Partial
(fortunately!)

What electrolyte abnormality is often seen with DiGeorge syndrome?

Hypocalcemia

Due to hypoparathyroidism (the parathyroid glands ordinarily located on the thyroid tissue also fail to form normally)

Which cardiac anomalies are most often present in DiGeorge syndrome patients?

1. **VSDs**
2. **Conotruncal abnormalities (things like tetralogy of Fallot, or transposition of the great vessels)**

If DiGeorge patients have mainly T cell abnormalities, what sort of infection(s) are they most at risk for?

(3)

1. **Fungi**
2. **Viruses**
3. **Opportunistic organisms, such as PCP**

(*P. jiroveci*, the cause of PCP is now considered a protozoan)

Sinus & pulmonary infections are common in a variety of immune deficiencies. If the vignette also mentions an elevated α1-fetoprotein, what is the disorder?

Ataxia – telangiectasia

What is the underlying problem in ataxia-telangiectasia?

Defective DNA strand repair, due to a mutation in the ATM gene

(there are several subtypes – some are unusually sensitive to radiation damage – important to know if ordering radiology evaluations!)

What is the main problem affecting daily life for ataxia-telangiectasia patients?

Neurological problems –
Especially cerebellar ataxia

How do children with ataxia-telangiectasia present?

**Ataxia first – in early childhood
Immune deficiency
Telangiectasias later**

The board gives you a photo item of an eye with telangiectasia on the bulbar conjunctiva (the conjunctiva over the sclera). What immune disorder are they probably showing you?

Ataxia-telangiectasia

How is the immune system affected in ataxia-telangiectasia?
  (2 main effects)

B & T cell counts are low & cell function is often not good

&

Hypogammaglobulinemia
(due to impaired class switching)

Is ataxia-telangiectasia commonly diagnosed in the first year of life?

No

A child more than one year old + ataxia + α 1-fetoprotein = what diagnosis?

Ataxia-telangiectasia

Long-term, what are the two most severe complication of ataxia telangiectasia?

High rate of malignancy, especially leukemia/lymphoma

&

Severe pulmonary infection

Bloom syndrome is a consequence of what enzyme deficiency?

BLM gene

(it codes for a helicase in the nuclear matrix of growing cells)

Bloom syndrome presents very similarly to what other DNA repair disorder?

Ataxia-telangiectasia

(the DNA repair defect is also very similar)

The main features of Bloom syndrome are _____?
  (4)

1. Short stature with microcephaly
2. Telangiectasia (sun-sensitive ones)
3. Immune deficiency
4. Early cancer development (especially leukemia)

Nijmegen breakage syndrome is rare, but tested on exams. What unusual combination of neuro-related findings occurs in this immunodeficiency syndrome?

Microcephaly

With

Normal IQ in early childhood (it later declines)

Nijmegen breakage syndrome, along with the closely related Berlin breakage syndrome, is considered to be a variant genetic disorder of what other DNA repair disorder?

Ataxia-telangiectasia variants

What malignancy are Nijmegen syndrome children likely to develop?

Lymphoid malignancies

What is the underlying problem in Nijmegen (breakage) syndrome?

Double-stranded DNA breaks are not repaired

(due to a missing protein)

Immune issues (both cellular & humoral) + normal IQ + small head = what disorder?

Nijmegen syndrome

Small platelets, and a low platelet count, are highly suggestive of what immune system disorder?

Wiskott-Aldrich syndrome

What triad is the core of Wiskott-Aldrich symptomatology?

- **Eczema**
- **Thrombocytopenia**
- **Frequent infections**

Mnemonic: Think of Buzz "Aldrin" (the astronaut) looking out from a space capsule with a runny nose, skin trouble, & bruising.

A boy who nearly exsanguinates after circumcision in the neonatal period is a boards example of what syndrome?

Wiskott-Aldrich

Wiskott-Aldrich syndrome kids are at increased risk for what malignancies?

Leukemia

&

Lymphoma

Wiskott-Aldrich patients have both B & T cells. How do they respond to vaccination?	**No adequate response** (they have difficulty making antigen specific antibodies)
How should Wiskott-Aldrich patients be treated if exposed to a dangerous infectious (especially if they have a history of serious infections)?	**IVIG**
What is currently the best overall treatment strategy for Wiskott-Aldrich syndrome patients?	**Bone marrow transplant** (matched sibling transplant 90 % successful currently)
What do you need to order, or instruct, to prepare the Wiskott-Aldrich patient for BMT? (2 orders, 1 instruction)	**IVIG** **Prophylactic antibiotics** **Avoidance of trauma-related bleeding**
At this point in history, what is the most common cause of death for Wiskott-Aldrich patients?	Infection (50 %) *(bleeding & malignancy make up about 25 % each)*
What is the expected life-span for a Wiskott-Aldrich patient?	Adolescence
In Wiskott-Aldrich patients with prominent eczematous skin findings, what do you expect to see on their lab work?	**Eosinophilia** & ↑ **IgE**
Bloody diarrhea in a very young infant who is found to have thrombocytopenia and eczema could be a presentation of _____ immune deficiency syndrome?	**Wiskott-Aldrich**
Splenectomy was sometimes suggested as a way to handle the thrombocytopenia of Wiskott-Aldrich. Why is this no longer recommended?	• Increased risk of sepsis!!! • Worsens humoral immunity • Makes patient even more vulnerable to encapsulated organisms (sepsis)

When B cells are missing or dysfunctional, what types of infections are most common?

Respiratory bacterial infections and chronic gut infections (including Giardia)

When immunoglobulins are not working properly, what types of bacteria are most likely to be problematic?

Encapsulated & pyogenic

What physical exam finding is a clue that a B cell immunodeficiency (meaning low numbers of B cells) may be present?

Absent or hypoplastic tonsils

What lab test is most crucial in detecting & identifying B cell problems?

Tests of "specific antibody formation" *(meaning response to a particular antigen)*

&

Ig production in various Ig classes

What is the other name for X-linked agammaglobulinemia?

Bruton (agammaglobulinemia)

What gene causes the problem in Bruton X-linked agammaglobulinemia?

BTK (on Xq22)

What is the underlying problem in Bruton agammaglobulinemia?

Bruton tyrosine kinase (BTK) is not made – it is necessary for B-cell maturity

What is the mainstay of treatment for X-linked agammaglobulinemia?

Monthly IVIG (to prevent infections)

How early should mainstay treatment for X-linked agammaglobulinemia be started?

Very early, 5 weeks is recommended

Earlier treatment is correlated with better outcomes

What vaccine must be especially avoided with Bruton patients?

Live (oral) polio virus vaccine, and ALL other live virus vaccines

Which immunoglobulin classes are low in Bruton?	**All of them (Bruton agammaglobulinemia, meaning "without")**
What unusual cell is sometimes found in the circulating blood of Bruton patients?	**B cell precursors**
Which infections are Bruton agammaglobulinemia patients especially vulnerable to?	**Respiratory tract infections with encapsulated bacteria**
Specifically, infections of which three parts of the body are often seen in Bruton?	**1. Sinuses 2. Ears 3. Lungs**
Classically, how does Bruton present?	**Boy with recurrent infections toward end of first year (transplacental maternal IgG gone)**
Will an X-linked agammaglobulinemia patient have improved immunity to a disease if an immunization is given?	**No – They don't make antibodies in response to antigen!**
Do X-linked agammaglobulinemia patients have antibodies to foreign blood groups?	**No – They don't make specific antibodies** *(they don't make any antibodies, at all!)*
Why do X-linked agammaglobulinemia patients often present at 6–9 months old?	**Because maternal antibodies disappear around that time**
Children with immunodeficiencies involving B cells are especially at risk for what GI infection?	**Chronic giardiasis**
What finding on physical exam of the lymphatic system suggests Bruton agammaglobulinemia?	Small tonsils or lymph nodes
Which immune disorder is entirely silent until the patient contracts EBV?	**X-linked Lymphoproliferative Disease** **(XLP)**

What is the other name for X-linked lymphoproliferative disease?	Duncan disease (named for the family in which it was first identified – 6 of 18 males in that family died due to XLP)

Mnemonic: Duncan in Shakespeare's MacBeth was a guy (X-linked). His troubles "proliferated" when he visited MacBeth, and was killed! |
What happens when an XLP patient contracts EBV?	**Polyclonal expansion of both T & B cell lines occurs →** **B cell lymphomas, aplastic anemia, fulminant hepatitis**
What are the most common causes of death among XLP patients? (2)	1. Hepatic necrosis (fulminant!) 2. Bone marrow failure
Do X-linked lymphoproliferative syndrome patients have immune system deficiencies prior to EBV infection?	**No**
Can XLP be prevented?	Yes – Bone marrow transplant can be done *before* EBV infection happens

(if you know the patient has the syndrome!) |
Why does bone marrow failure occur in XLP?	Both the liver damage & bone marrow failure result from hemophagocytic lymphohistiocytosis (a severe overactivation of the T-cell and macrophage systems)
If an X-linked lymphoproliferative patient survives the initial EBV episode, are there any long-term problems?	Yes – They have antibody deficiency & risk of malignancy
When do infants begin to produce their own IgG?	2–3 months old

When is it normal for infants' IgG level to drop? ("physiological nadir")

4–6 months old

What is "transient hypogammaglobulinemia of infancy?"

Low IgG in an infant for an unusually long time

What do we call the "normal" IgG level decline between 4 and 6 months of age?

"Physiological" hypogammaglobulinemia

What is the usual course of transient hypogammaglobulinemia of infancy?

Asymptomatic, with return to normal levels between 2 and 6 years old

Are the B or T cells abnormal in children with transient hypogammaglobulinemia of infancy?

No – The IgG amount produced is just lower than expected

Is IVIG needed for infants with transient hypogammaglobulinemia of infancy?

Usually not, but the child should be monitored for infection, and can require treatment

IgG has four types. Deficiency of which type is sometimes associated with frequent sinus infections?

IgG <u>2</u>

IgG 2 deficiency is associated with what types of frequent infections? (4)

1. Sinusitis
2. Pneumonia
3. Otitis media
4. Bronchitis

If a child has IgG 2 subclass deficiency, what do you expect their overall IgG level to be?

Normal or borderline low

If a child with a normal immune system has frequent infections, what do you expect to see on his or her IgG levels?

High IgG

Although it is not common practice in real life, it is fine to look for IgG 2 subclass deficiency on the boards by ordering what test?

IgG subclass levels (in response to a specific antigen, like *S. pneumo*)

If you suspect a complement deficiency as a cause of immune problems, what is the initial screening test?

CH50 or AP50

(CH = classic hemolytic pathway)
(AP = alternative hemolytic pathway)

Which patients should you automatically suspect of having a complement deficiency?

Meningococcus patients
(*Neisseria meningococcus*)

(20 % have a complement deficiency!)

If a meningococcus patient has a complement deficiency, which parts of the complement system are likely to be the problem?

"Terminal" or late components that form the "MAC" attack complex
(C5–9)

How does inheritance work for complement genes?

Autosomal "codominant"

What does autosomal codominant mean, clinically?

Both alleles of the gene are active & expressed

Your patient has an enzyme-related genetic disorder with autosomal codominant inheritance. One allele is normal, but the other is nonfunctional. What does this mean, in general terms, for the enzyme production?

Approximately 50 % of normal enzyme activity should result

(both genes are expressed, but only one produces a functional enzyme)

If your patient is heterozygous for a complement deficiency, will he or she have problems with immune function?

No –
But they may have more autoimmune disease

If you had to choose the one part of the complement cascade that is most critical, which part would it be?

C3

(Does most activation, and is important in both the classical & alternative pathway)

Over time, do patients with complement deficiencies tend to get better or worse?

Better
(As antibody memory responses are developed to most antigens)

Frequent abdominal pain combined with extremity or facial swelling = what complement disorder?

Hereditary angioedema

What causes hereditary angioedema (Types I & II)?

C1 esterase inhibitor is missing or low

Why is it a problem if you can't inhibit complement C1?

C1 inhibitor also inhibits bradykinin – When bradykinin runs wild, things swell up

Why would C1 inhibitor deficient patients have gut pain?

Gut wall edema develops due to overactive bradykinin

Can an acute episode of hereditary angioedema in the gut result in any serious consequences?

Yes –
Sometimes, there is enough third spacing due to the leaky tissues involved that fluid resuscitation can be necessary

(*& occasionally unnecessary abdominal surgery, if the belly pain is interpreted as an acute abdomen!*)

What is the life-threatening aspect of hereditary angioedema?

Airway swelling!!

When C1 is not inhibited, what other aspects of the complement cascade will be affected?

C2 & C4 are chronically used up

How is hereditary angioedema inherited?

Autosomal dominant mainly (Types I & II)

(A third type has now been described, seen only in females, but the inheritance is not entirely clear and its mechanism is a bit different)

A hereditary angioedema episode looks a lot like an acute allergic reaction. Are steroids, H1/H2 blockers, or epinephrine helpful?

No

Which uncommon medication is helpful in an episode of hereditary angioedema, although it takes *2 days* to work?

ε-Aminocaproic acid

(brand name Amicar®)

In an acute attack of airway angioedema, what is the most important aspect of management?

Protect the airway – Intubate *before* it closes

Give C1 inhibitor replacement

(Fresh frozen plasma (FFP) can be used if specific C1 inhibitor replacement is not available, because FFP also contains the inhibitory enzyme)

Do hereditary angioedema patients "swell up all over?"

No –
The swelling is localized
(although there might be multiple areas of localized swelling)

If hives are present (a wheal or wheal & flare skin reaction) on a patient you suspect has hereditary angioedema (HAE), do the hives make the HAE diagnosis more or less likely?

Less likely

Should a patient with HAE limit their activity in any way?

Yes –
Avoid contact sports because trauma is a common trigger for acute attacks

(Surgery & dental work can also trigger attacks, for the same reason)

Are preventive medication regimens used in the treatment of hereditary angioedema?

Yes –
Antifibrinolytics are sometimes used for long-term prophylaxis in children (efficacy not really clear)

&

Attenuated androgens (at the lowest possible dose – they affect C1 esterase levels)

How is HAE type III different from types I & II, in terms of its mechanism?

C1 esterase inhibitor level is normal

Levels of bradykinin rise (possibly due to an overactive, different, enzyme)

It is affected by estrogen levels

What is unusual about the epidemiology of HAE Type III?

It is seen only in females

In general, live vaccines (viral or bacterial) should not be given to what groups of children? (3)

1. Immune suppressed
2. Immune deficiencies
3. Bone marrow transplant patients (if their immune system is not yet reconstituted)

Which commonly encountered vaccinations (in the USA or other countries) are live?

1. BCG (tuberculosis)
2. OPV (oral polio)
3. MMR (measles, mumps, rubella)
4. Varicella vaccine (chicken pox)

Is it alright for the household contact of an immunocompromised child to receive the MMR or varicella vaccines?

Yes

Is it alright for household contacts of an immunocompromised child to receive the oral polio virus vaccine?

No –
The virus is shed in the gut/feces

Most flu vaccine is fine for household contacts of immunodeficient patients. Which type is *not*?

Intranasal
Influenza
Vaccine
(it's live)

Smallpox vaccine has recently become a topic again due to bioterrorism concerns. Is this a live or "killed" vaccine?

Live

Which patients should not receive smallpox vaccine? (3)

Immunodeficient
Pregnant
Atopic dermatitis patients

What is the problem with giving atopic dermatitis patients the smallpox vaccine?

They are more likely to "lose control" of cutaneous viruses and develop a serious reaction or infection

(same as is seen with herpes simplex infections in atopic dermatitis patients – although that's not a vaccine)

Why shouldn't contacts of immunodeficient patients receive smallpox vaccination?
(household or healthcare contacts)

The virus is shed from the skin

When can an immunocompromised patient safely come in contact with someone recently smallpox immunized?

When the skin lesion is healed

(about 3 weeks)

If a child is taking oral steroids, is it alright to give live vaccines?

No –
Unless the dose is low, <2 mg/kg per day

How long should you wait after a child has stopped taking oral steroids to give a live vaccine?
(unless it was a very short 3–5-day course)

At least 1 month

Are inhaled steroids as much of a concern, in terms of vaccination with live attenuated viruses?

No

Caveat: Clinical experience indicates that it is alright, although the data is not sufficient to give a final answer to this question.

What about the use of nasal (not inhaled, but nasal) or topical steroids for vaccination with live attenuated virus vaccines?

Same answer –
Clinical experience indicates that it is well tolerated

Children with HIV are immunocompromised. Should they receive the MMR?	Yes, but to be eligible: Must have CD4+ T cell counts ≥ 15 % of expected normal value for at least 6 months if ≤ 5 years old. Children older than 5 years must meet the 15 % criterion & have ≥ 200 CD4+ T cell count Although it is live, the benefit is bigger than the risk of problems from the vaccine
Is it alright to give the varicella vaccine to very young HIV+ children?	If they are not severely immunocompromised or very symptomatic & T cell count is ≥ 15 % of expected (applies children at least 12 months old)
What is recommended for HIV+ children who are more than 8 years old, and still in need of varicella vaccine?	It is okay if the CD4+ T cell count is ≥ 200 cells/μL
Which combination vaccination should you be sure not to give to your immunocompromised patients?	The combined measles, mumps, rubella, and varicella vaccine (ProQuad®)
Should the OPV vaccine (oral polio) get anywhere near an HIV+ child?	No
Mold is sometimes an allergen. In a northern climate, what will you often observe with mold allergies?	Improvement during cold and dry seasons
In southern climates, what pattern do you expect to see for mold allergies?	Usually year round

Many patients complain of seasonal allergies in the spring. Which pollens are at their peak in the spring?	Tree pollens
Fall allergies are likely due to what type of plant pollen?	Weeds!!
Why do patients with allergies sometimes have daytime or nighttime coughing?	Postnasal drip
If both parents have allergies, what is the probability that the child will also?	About 60 %
Frequent sneezing, clear runny nose, and itchy eyes & nose suggest what diagnosis?	Allergic rhinitis/conjunctivitis
Do allergies cause fevers?	Generally not
If a patient's symptoms respond to antihistamine treatment, the cause of the symptoms is probably _____?	Allergy
If a cough responds to bronchodilator therapy, it is likely that patient has _____?	Reactive airway disease (which may, or may not be, asthma)
If a patient's allergy symptoms flare up with vacuuming, he or she is probably allergic to what substances?	Dust/dust mites
In your boards vignette, if a patient's allergy symptoms flare when he or she enters a *barn*, the problem is likely to be what allergen?	Mold
Early summer allergy flares are usually due to which pollens?	Grass

What is the order for the plants producing the most pollen – spring, early summer, and fall?	Tree Grass Weed Mnemonic: Think of them going from tallest to shortest
Dark circles under the eyes are a sign of _____?	**Nasal congestion (allergic or other causes)**
What is a "nasal salute?"	Rubbing the nose upward with the hand to relieve both itching & nasal mucous – The nose sticks up a little & may develop a crease due to frequent rubbing
What are "Dennie-Morgan" lines?	**Wrinkles below the eyes (often goes with atopic conditions)**
Why is mouth breathing common in allergy sufferers?	Tonsil & adenoid enlargement
Chronic postnasal discharge leads to what physical finding on the posterior pharynx?	**"Cobblestone" appearance**
In allergy, should conjunctivitis be unilateral or bilateral?	**Bilateral!**
Asthma can be exacerbated by allergies. Should asthmatics have clubbing on physical exam?	No – O_2 delivery is not chronically compromised
What physical finding (change) is common in the chests of those with long-term asthma?	Increased chest AP diameter (due to chronic air trapping – barrel-shaped chest)
How long must a patient be off diphenhydramine for skin allergy testing to be valid?	**72 h** **(longer for long-acting antihistamines)** *(Only H1 blockers have this effect!)*
Explain the two types of skin testing for allergies?	**1. Epicutaneous – skin is pricked while a drop of antigen extract sits on it** **2. Intradermal – allergen extract is injected**

What is a positive reaction to a skin allergy test?	**Wheal & flare**
Why does a wheal develop in positive allergy tests?	**Type 1 (local) hypersensitivity** (Remember, this means that allergen has bound to preformed IgE, causing mast cell degranulation)
Will antihistamines block type 1 hypersensitivity reactions?	**Yes**
Will steroids block type 1 hypersensitivity reactions?	**No** **(May block type 4 delayed response, though)**
What CBC finding is often present in atopic individuals?	↑ **eosinophils** (>5 % is high)
Which immunoglobulin is often elevated in atopic individuals?	**IgE**
If a patient's skin allergy test is negative for a particular antigen, can you be confident that he or she is *not* allergic to that substance?	**Generally, yes –** **the results much be correlated with clinical history, as always**
What is the significance of a positive response to a skin allergen test?	Suggestive of allergy, but not conclusive
What is the in vitro (blood) testing system for allergies called?	**Antigen-specific IgE immunoassay** **(The older type of blood-based in vitro testing for allergy is called RAST, which stands for "RadioAllergoSorbent Testing." This term is still used at times, but current preferred methods do not use radiation, so it is not accurate.)**
What are the advantages of specific IgE testing for allergies?	**1. No risk of anaphylaxis** **2. Histamine medications will not affect the results**

Do home air filtration systems help with dust mite allergy?	**No** (Not many of their allergens are airborne)
Do HEPA air filters help with decreasing pet-related allergens?	Yes
What is the best way to decrease the allergen burden from a pet?	**Get rid of the pet** *Remember that pet allergens are still present for about 6 months to 1 year afterwards, though!!*
What is the main side effect of antihistamine use?	**Sedation**
Why are more recently developed antihistamines less sedating? (2)	1. They are more H1 receptor specific 2. They don't cross the blood-brain barrier very well
At what point in the allergy cycle are antihistamines most effective?	<u>Before</u> exposure
Do antihistamines prevent mast cell degranulation, if given before allergen exposure?	**No –** **Mast cells degranulate when IgE molecules on their surface cross-link due to antigen showing up!**
Are medications available that prevent mast cell degranulation? If yes, what are they called?	• Yes • Mast cell stabilizers (for example, Cromolyn)
When are mast cell degranulation medications helpful, in the allergy cycle?	<u>Before</u> exposure
How can steroids be helpful in allergic response?	Reduce late-phase symptoms
How are steroids mainly used in the management of non-acute allergies?	Intranasally, to reduce allergic rhinitis
Do intranasal steroids have systemic effects?	Supposedly not (most existing data indicates they do not have any significant systemic effects, but there is some controversy about this)

If exposure prevention & medications are not effective management for allergies, what is the next step?

Allergen immunotherapy

How long does immunotherapy usually take to work?

1–2 *years*

How is immunotherapy for allergy performed?

SubQ injections of increasing amounts of the offending allergen are given over time

Is immunotherapy indicated for patients who have systemic reactions to hymenoptera stings (like wheezing or hypotension)?

Yes – Regardless of age

What sorts of systemic reactions to hymenoptera venom are common in children?

Skin
   &
Respiratory

(cardiovascular reactions are relatively uncommon in children – more common in adults)

Why do allergies to seasonal allergens like pollens present at a later age than year-round exposures like dust mites?

Repeated exposure over multiple seasons is needed to develop an allergy, in most cases

At what age does seasonal allergy usually present?

Age 5 years or later

If the first phase of the allergic response is mast cell degranulation, what causes the second and chronic phases?

T helper cells
   &
Eosinophils

Nasal polyps go along with allergic rhinitis in adolescent and adults. What do nasal polyps suggest in young children?

CF

(Cystic fibrosis)

If you're thinking of allergic rhinitis as a diagnosis, what microscopic finding in the nasal secretions would help to support your diagnosis?

Eosinophils

What option is available for treating allergic conjunctivitis?

Ocular drops that stabilize mast cells & also have antihistamine properties

(e.g., olopatadine)

Which congenital anomalies make latex allergy more likely than usual? (2)

Neural tube defects (including spina bifida)

&

Urological abnormalities

Multiple surgeries in infancy/early childhood are the strongest risk factor for which allergy?

Latex allergy

What molecules is the latex allergic patient usually reacting to?

Hevein (a protein from the commercial rubber tree, *Hevea brasiliensis*)

(Subtypes Hev b 1 to Hev b 6 are mainly involved – there are 11 Hev b subtypes in total)

If you want to do skin testing for latex allergy, what will limit your ability to do this?

Good skin test reagents are not available for latex

Prior allergy to which four types of fruit or nuts increases the probability of latex allergy?

1. Bananas
2. Kiwi
3. Avocado
4. Chestnuts

A PCN allergic patient is more likely to react to which antibiotic – imipenem or aztreonam?

Imipenem

Mnemonic: It has a lot of "i's" and "p's" like penicillin.

PCN allergic patients (by self-report or documented incident) were initially thought to have 50 % cross-reactivity with carbapenem antibiotics like imipenem. *Current data suggests that cross-reactivity is about 10 %.*

Aztreonam is a monobactam, with very little cross-reactivity to penicillins

PCN-allergic patients have what likelihood of allergic reaction to a cephalosporin?

5–10 %
(or 1 in 10–20 PCN-allergic patients)

If a patient is having an allergic reaction to a currently prescribed medication, what is the first thing you must do?

Stop the drug!

If an acute allergic reaction is occurring, involving airway or blood pressure issues, how should you treat the patient?
(3)

1. Epinephrine first!
2. Steroids
3. H1 & H2 blockers

If a patient has neurosyphilis, and is PCN-allergic, what should you do to treat the infection?

Desensitize

&

Give PCN

(neurosyphilis does not have to occur far into the disease – it can appear in young patients)

If a pregnant patient is found to have syphilis, but is also PCN-allergic, what should you do?

Desensitize

&

Give PCN

In general terms, what is PCN desensitization?	Giving a very small dose of penicillin orally or IV, followed by gradually increasing doses given in rapid succession (e.g., 15 min apart, but for some agents intervals are longer), until a full dose is tolerated
If you have desensitized a patient for administration of a needed medication, will you need to desensitize the patient again if another illness requires the same medication?	Yes – Desensitization is usually good for only one episode of treatment (The patient loses desensitization after missing 1–2 sequential doses of the medication)
Is desensitization successful with all types of hypersensitivity reactions?	**No –** **Usually just type 1** **(IgE mediated)**
How can you tell whether a drug reaction is likely to be an IgE-mediated reaction or not? (2)	1. It should occur within an hour of so of giving the drug 2. Wheal & flare reaction is suggestive
Severe skin reactions to drugs, such as Stevens-Johnson syndrome & toxic epidermal necrolysis, usually develop how long after a drug is given?	>72 h
Is skin testing for drug allergies helpful in determining a cause?	**Yes,** **But only PCN testing is validated with good sensitivity and specificity**
If allergy to PCN is suspected, what do you need to order to be sure you've done a thorough job?	Major *and minor* penicillin determinants
What hematological reaction sometimes occurs with drug administration and immune response?	Hemolytic anemia
If a patient has a history of significant allergies or anaphylaxis, what should you prescribe?	**The Epi-Pen!**

Do atopic children have an increased risk of anaphylaxis?

Yes, but only for anaphylaxis triggered by:
Latex
Exercise &
Food

What broad medication classes most commonly cause anaphylaxis?

NSAIDs
Antibiotics

&

Anesthetics
(especially local anesthetics & neuromuscular blocking agents used in general anesthesia)

Which foods are most likely to produce anaphylaxis?
　(4 groups)

Nuts – peanuts & tree nuts
Milk & eggs
Fish & shellfish
Grains – specifically soy & wheat

(90 % of US cases of food anaphylaxis result from these four groups)

When a patient has a reaction that looks like anaphylaxis, but the problem was *not IgE mediated,* what is it called?

Anaphylact<u>oid</u> – also known as pseudoanaphylaxis

If you want to verify whether a reaction was anaphylactic, what lab test can you send?

Tryptase –
If sent within the first few hours after the reaction begins

(confirms mast cell degranulation)

Do all anaphylaxis patients have skin findings?

No –
But most have either urticaria or flushing

Will some anaphylaxis patients complain of GI symptoms?

Yes –
Don't let that fool you!

What are the main problems in anaphylaxis?

1. Vasodilation & vascular leakiness → hypotension
2. Smooth muscle contraction in the lung + leaky lung capillaries → respiratory compromise

Some reactions to food are not caused by immune or allergic mechanisms. What are the other two common reasons?	1. Enzyme deficiency 2. Toxin in the food
True food allergy affects what percentage of the population younger than 5 years old?	**~5–10 %**
The most common symptoms of food allergy are _____ & _____?	**1. Skin reactions (itching, edema, urticaria)** **2. Upper respiratory symptoms**
What GI complaints go along with food allergy?	**Nausea, vomiting, abdominal pain**
Are wheat, soy, & cow's milk enterocolitis generally IgE mediated?	**No**
Which food allergies are usually lifelong problems?	Nuts & Shellfish/fish
Does food allergy cause chronic (allergic) rhinitis?	**No** **(That comes from inhaled allergens)**
If skin testing for a food allergen is negative, what should you conclude?	**It's *not* the problem –** **But in unusual cases further testing could be needed, if the clinical history is compelling**
If a patient has been previously diagnosed with a food allergy, should you assume the food allergy is real?	**No –** **Food allergy is frequently overdiagnosed** (about 1/3 will be true allergies)
Can a true type 1 hypersensitivity reaction occur without prior exposure?	**No –** B cells must be presented with the antigen, and then generate IgE, so that the reaction can occur right away, upon exposure to the antigen. The first exposure is required for generation of the IgE.

How long does it usually take for a type 3 serum sickness reaction to develop?	**1–3 weeks**
How does a type III reaction happen?	**Antigen-antibody complexes form, are deposited in tissue, and activate complement**
Is IgE involved in serum sickness (type III)?	No
Which immunoglobulins are involved in serum sickness (type III hypersensitivity reactions)?	IgG Or IgM
Do type III reactions require prior exposure to the antigen?	**No**
Which tissues are mainly affected in serum sickness? **(3 tissues)**	**Joints** **Vessel walls** **Renal glomeruli** (GI & pulmonary also affected)
What do serum sickness patients usually complain of? (3 groups)	• Skin swelling, erythema, edema • Joint & muscle pain • GI complaints
What urine finding is expected in serum sickness?	Proteinuria (may also find microscopic hematuria & hyaline casts)
How is serum sickness treated?	**Antihistamines (for itch)** **NSAIDS (for joints)** **Steroids PRN (for severe cases)**
What is the usual course for serum sickness?	**Spontaneous resolution after 7–10 days**
How does serum sickness differ from immediate hypersensitivity reactions?	1. Later onset (1–3 weeks) 2. IgG or IgM + complement mediated 3. Less acute

What typically gets serum sickness started?	1. Heterologous serum proteins (proteins from serum of other species) such as some antitoxins & antivenoms 2. Medications (especially antibiotics, in children, cefaclor in particular) 3. Biologic agents (e.g., monoclonal antibodies)
A neonate is brought to your office because the umbilical stump has not fallen off. The baby is nearly 4 weeks old. What is the problem, and why didn't the stump fall off?	• **Leukocyte adhesion defect (type 1)** • **The leukocytes can't attack the stump properly, to weaken it so it will fall off**
A child has a high neutrophil count, but problems with frequent infections & abscesses. What is the likely problem?	**LAD (leukocyte adhesion defect type 1)** (Type 2 is very rare & presents the same + mr and developmental delay)
Which immune cells need adhesion molecules most to function well?	Phagocytes
Why would children with leukocyte adhesion defect have a high neutrophil count?	If neutrophils don't have adhesion molecules, they can't stick to things – that means they can't get stopped to crawl out of the blood vessel *So the count in the blood is higher than normal!*
A patient presents with *multiple abscesses – but no erythema, heat, or pain* associated with them. The child is 9 years old, and has a history notable for *staphylococcal pneumonia & osteomyelitis*. What is the disorder, and what will you see on labs?	• **Hyper IgE syndrome** • **Eosinophilia & ↑ IgE** (also known as Job's syndrome)
Abscesses that don't generate pain, heat, or redness are referred to as _____ _____?	**"Cold" abscesses** (Hyper IgE syndrome)

A chest x-ray is shown along with a vignette about a child who has *recurrent staph infections*, coarse facies, *eczema*, and *eosinophilia*. What is the chest X-ray likely to show, and why?

Pneumatoceles –
They are trying to tell you this is hyper IgE syndrome, and the child has had Staph pneumonia

(could also show a lung abscess)

What do you need to know about Chediak-Higashi syndrome?
   (3 items)

1. It involves immune dysfunction
2. Oculocutaneous albinism is a buzzword for it (not fully lacking in pigment, but light skin & irises, blond or silvery hair)
3. Big granules are common in immune cells

What is the prognosis for Chediak-Higashi patients?

Poor without treatment –

But bone marrow transplant can be curative for the immune system problems

Chediak-Higashi patients who survive into later childhood or adulthood often develop significant & disabling problems in which body system?

Neurological –
Peripheral and central nervous system degeneration, including intellectual disability & movement-related changes (of many different sorts)

What is the problem in Chediak-Higashi syndrome?

Storage organelles (e.g., lysosomes & melanosomes) don't form or function properly –
That's why there are abnormally large granules in the immune cells

(material is stuck inside lysosomes that can't fuse to other things properly)

What recessively inherited disorder presents with *recurrent infections, partial oculocutaneous albinism, & big granules* in blood smear of immune cells?

Chediak-Higashi, of course!

Mnemonic: Think of some Japanese kids playing a defective version of "Pacman®," called Chediakman! In this game, the Chediakman attacks but can't eat any of the game pieces.

(The Japanese kids are to help you recognize the second part of the name "Higashi")

Which immune disorder is X-linked, causes problems with NADPH oxidase, and results in multiple infections with catalase-positive bacteria?

Chronic granulomatous disease

Which important bacteria are catalase-positive?
(five of them – Four start with "s")

1. *Staph aureus*
2. Staph epidermidis
3. Serratia maracescens
4. Salmonella
5. *E. coli*

Why does it matter if a cell is NADPH oxidase deficient?

Phagocytes use it to generate H_2O_2 – One of the main ways to kill ingested bacteria

Which immune cells have a problem in chronic granulomatous disease?

Phagocytes

Why can chronic granulomatous disease patients kill some bacteria, and not others?

Bacteria produce their own H_2O_2 – Some bacteria can get rid of what they produce and others can't
Those that can't "commit suicide" by producing their own H_2O_2 inside the phagocyte!

How do you test for chronic granulomatous disease?

Historically nitroblue tetrazolium reduction (NBT) –
Deficient leukocytes can't reduce the NBT dye

Now tested with dihydrorhodamine oxidation test (DHR) –
DHR is a flow cytometry test that measures fluorescence from the oxidation of the DHR to the rhodamine 123 molecule – if the neutrophils can't oxidize, fluorescent molecules are not produced

A child <2 years old presents with *recurrent abscesses* and *draining lymphadenitis*. On exam, he has *hepatosplenomegaly*. What immune disorder should you consider?

Chronic granulomatous disease

How is chronic granulomatous disease inherited?

X-linked

Or

Autosomal recessive

How is chronic granulomatous disease treated?

Prophylactic antibiotics and antifungals (usually TMP/SMX & itraconazole)

&

IFN-gamma

What is the relationship between complement deficiencies and lupus?

Both systemic lupus & discoid lupus (skin only) are associated with complement deficiency

(C2, 3, 4, & C1q, R, S – C1q deficiency is the strongest genetic risk factor for development of systemic lupus)

Chapter 3
Selected Hematology and Oncology Topics: Hamartomas vs. Teratomas

Hamartoma? What is that?

The definition of a hamartoma is a focal overgrowth of cells and tissues that are *native to the organ in which they are growing*. The overgrowth is made up of **normal cells** growing with **abnormal architecture**.

The line separating hamartomas from benign neoplasms is not clear to anyone. Some growths are simply referred to as hamartomas by tradition. Examples of growths that can be considered hamartomas include:

Hemangiomas
Adenomas
Rhabdomyomas

Hamartomas are thought to be a developmental anomaly (mistake in growth), and are most common in infancy and childhood. Some regress on their own.

Think of a "hammer-shaped" mass of cells inside an organ to remember "hammer-toma" – they are cells that would normally be there, just not so many of them.

Teratoma – Does this have to do with the plantation in *"Gone With The Wind?"*

Unfortunately, there is nothing very Scarlett O'Hara about teratomas. Scarlett was the right age, though, to develop one!

(For those of you who aren't fans, the plantation was called "Tara.")

Teratomas are tumors composed of a variety of parenchymal cells. Most typically, the tissue types represent all three embryonal germ layers (endoderm, ectoderm, and mesoderm). This often makes them easy to see radiologically, as they frequently contain unusual structures like hair and teeth.

© Springer Science+Business Media New York 2016
C.M. Houser, *Pediatric Tricky Topics, Volume 2*,
DOI 10.1007/978-1-4939-3109-5_3

Most teratomas develop on midline or reproductive structures. There are two peaks in the appearance of teratomas – around 2 years old and around 20 years old.

Are teratomas benign?

It depends. The aggressiveness of the tumor is determined by the level of differentiation of its cells. Many are benign.

Chapter 4
General Hematology and Oncology Question and Answer Items

What is the Mentzer Index?	**A quick calculation that helps you identify iron-deficiency anemia vs. thalassemia minor**
How do you calculate the Mentzer Index?	**MCV/RBC count**
How do you interpret the Mentzer Index?	**<13 means thalassemia** **>13 means iron deficiency** (iron-deficiency anemia is <u>much</u> more common, so it gets the bigger numbers)
What is the *most prevalent* sort of hematological disorder in the USA?	**Iron-deficiency anemia**
What happens to the total iron-binding capacity (TIBC) in iron-deficiency anemia?	It goes up (the body is trying to find more iron)
What happens to serum ferritin in iron-deficiency anemia?	It goes down (because it is a type of iron in the blood)
If iron is provided to a patient with iron-deficiency anemia, when would you expect the reticulocyte count to start going up?	A week (or a little less)

© Springer Science+Business Media New York 2016
C.M. Houser, *Pediatric Tricky Topics, Volume 2*,
DOI 10.1007/978-1-4939-3109-5_4

Will the hemoglobin increase before or after the reticulocytes start to go up?	After (Think of the reticulocytes bringing the hemoglobin out into the circulation – that's why the hemoglobin *can't* go up until their numbers increase)
When your patient reaches a normal hemoglobin, and has normal red blood cell parameters, should you discontinue the iron and switch to dietary strategies?	No – Continue iron supplementation for 6–8 weeks to replete body stores
Lead poisoning interferes with which two enzymes in the heme-synthesis pathway (mainly)?	Ferrochelatase & gamma-ALA-D
Both lead poisoning and thalassemia minor can cause basophilic stippling. What differentiates the thalassemia cells?	Thalassemia has "target" cells, too
What should you expect for the RBC count with alpha thalassemia trait?	High or normal
What should you expect for the RBC count with lead toxicity or iron deficiency?	It goes down, of course (That's why they call it anemia, right?)
Which hemoglobin will be elevated on the electrophoresis of an alpha thalassemia trait patient?	A2
How can you diagnose sideroblastic anemia?	Bone marrow evaluation *only!*
How common is sideroblastic anemia in kids?	Rare!
A positive Coombs test means your patient's anemia is due to what general cause?	Immune system (autoimmune for SLE) (isoimmune for Rh or ABO)

Spherocytosis patients have a problem with spectrin and RBC cell membranes. What special complications are they likely to develop?

- **Gallstones very young**
- **Hemolytic & aplastic crises with infections**

Which medications are linked to the development of megaloblastic anemia in children?

- Dilantin
- Methotrexate
- Bactrim

(It's DuMB to get a medication MegaloBlastic anemia – might help you remember the drugs involved)

The classic blood smear for aplastic anemia is . . .?

Normocytic, normochromic, low retic count

(sudden onset problems with RBCs are generally normochromic, normocytic, because that's what is normally produced!)

If a patient has short stature and completely normal blood cell lines, except for an aplastic anemia, what diagnosis should you think of?

Diamond-Blackfan

What is the treatment for transient erythroblastopenia of childhood?

Time – most disorders with transient in the name resolve on their own

Which patient group most often develops transient erythroblastopenia of childhood?

1–4-year-olds
(Also seen in the first year, especially after 6 months of age)

What is the usually cited trigger for a bout of transient erythroblastopenia of childhood?

Viral illness
(of course, as with other virus-associated disorders, it is not clear whether viral illnesses actually cause it, or just happen to occur in lots of patients as a coincidence)

If you see a newborn or preemie with hemolysis, what nutritional cause should you consider?

Vitamin E deficiency

What is the underlying pathological process in leukemia?	Clonal proliferation of an abnormal cell line
Why do leukemia patients develop problems with anemia and bone marrow?	The abnormal clonal cells crowd the normal cells out of space in the marrow
What percentage of leukemia in children is acute lymphoblastic leukemia (ALL)?	**70 %**
What is a new name for acute myelogenous leukemia (AML)?	Acute non-lymphoblastic leukemia (ANLL)
How common is chronic myelogenous leukemia in children?	2–3 % of leukemias (the rest are ANLL aka AML, or ALL)
What is the importance of having a "CALLA (CD10)-positive" ALL?	**Very good prognosis** (Calla lilies are pretty, so it's a good thing to be Calla+)
Which ALL presents with a mediastinal mass in school-aged children?	T cell ALL – Easy to treat!
Which ALL is most aggressive & most rare (fortunately)?	Mature B cell ALL
Most ALL falls into what general subtype?	Pre-B ALL (Easiest ALL to treat!)
In the French-American-British (FAB) classification scheme for AML, which types have Auer rods in the abnormal cells?	M1 & M2 (all of the subtypes start with "M")
Which FAB type of AML occurs more often in trisomy 21 patients?	M7 (megakaryocytic) $7 \times 3 = 21$ Classification is 7 trisomy is 3 Particular trisomy involved is 21!

Which type of AML, in the FAB scheme, can be treated with vitamin A?
(also known as trans-retinoic acid)

M3 (promyelocytic)

What tests should you do when you are initially screening for a suspected leukemia?

CBC and diff

What tests will you need to do to confirm a diagnosis of leukemia, if your initial screen is worrisome?

Bone marrow aspirate & biopsy

When is the likelihood of DIC highest for leukemia patients?

At presentation –
10 % of patients *present* with DIC

When is tumor lysis syndrome most likely to occur in a patient with leukemia?

When treatment is first started

Trisomy 21 patients are at increased risk for leukemia. How much is their risk of ALL increased?

About 20×

Which very unusual form of AML are trisomy 21 patients much more likely to develop than most children?

M7 or acute megakaryoblastic leukemia (AMKL) –
500× increased risk!

What is unusual about the age of onset for AML in patients with trisomy 21?

It is younger –
Average onset about 2 years & most present before age 5

(general population average age at presentation 7.5 years)

Overall, what percentage of trisomy 21 patients will develop some type of leukemia?

2–3 %

Trisomy 21 patients are very unlikely to develop what general sort of malignancies?

Solid malignancies

Which immunodeficiency disorders put the patient at increased risk for leukemia?
(also at risk for lymphoma)

- **Wiskott-Aldrich**
- **Agammaglobulinemia**
- **SCID syndrome**

(Picture a dog with a runny nose and eyes because he is immunodeficient who WAGs his tail so hard he SCIDs)

Which genetic syndromes increase a patient's risk of leukemia?

- **Trisomy 21 (of course)**
- **Fanconi's anemia**
- **Bloom syndrome**
- **Ataxia telangiectasia**

(To remember the last three, think of a blood smear that looks like it's "blooming" with FAAT, because it's all white, due to the leukemic cells)

If you are treating ALL, how long should your initial attempt at induction last?

4 weeks

When you have completed the usual induction course, what do you need to check, to know how to proceed with treatment?

Bone marrow aspirate & CSF

What percentage of patients with ALL will have a successful induction course in just 4 weeks?

90 %

How important is it to check the leukemic cells for chromosomal translocations?

**Very important –
Specific translocations change treatment and prognosis**

(several worsen the prognosis, but some also improve it)

What is the DNA index for leukemic cells?

A ratio of chromosome number in the leukemic cells to the normal chromosome number, 46
(it is a measure of how much DNA is active in the cell)

Which is better, a lot of active DNA or not very much? Why?

Lots is better – if the cell's DNA is very active, then it will be very vulnerable to chemo agents

How can you remember which is better for the DNA index – a big number or a smaller number?	Bigger is better, because it means that the DNA takes up more of the cell's space (therefore it's more active than small, coiled, DNA)
Which other term is often used & means essentially the same thing as the DNA index?	The "hyperdiploidy" level of the abnormal cells
What is the important cutoff number for the DNA index in ALL?	**1.16 – less than 1.16 is *high risk***
What is the cutoff number for WBC count in ALL that means the patient is at high risk?	**>50,000**
If you had ALL, what would you want your WBC count to be?	**<50,000 (standard risk)**
What percentage of ALL patients are in complete remission 5 years after treatment is completed?	Around 85 % (they are probably cured)
How do the success rates for ALL compare to those for AML?	AML is worse *(overall long-term survival for pediatric patients is about 50 %, though – better for lower risk patients with matched bone marrow transplants)*
What is the mainstay of treatment for AML, in general?	Bone marrow transplant after first remission is induced (induction success rate is 70 %)
Which type of bone marrow transplantation is most often done?	**Allogeneic (HLA compatible, but genetically not identical)**
Autologous transplant means that the transplanted cells came from _____ ?	Patient's own stem cells
How do you determine how vulnerable to infectious agents a neutropenic patient will be?	Calculate the ANC (absolute neutrophil count)

In case you've forgotten, how do you calculate the ANC?	From the differential, add up the neutrophil and band count, then multiply that percentage by the total white count
What is a respectable ANC, meaning that your patient is at little risk of bacterial infection?	>1,000
How fast do you need to get antibiotics into a febrile neutropenic patient?	Emergently!
What is the main determinant of whether a patient will develop acute tumor lysis syndrome?	Amount of tumor – the more tumor there is, the greater the likelihood
Which two types of white cell cancers are most notorious for generating acute tumor lysis syndrome?	ALL & NHL (not the National Hockey League – Non-Hodgkin Lymphoma!)
Should you stop chemotherapy if a patient develops acute tumor lysis syndrome?	Yes – until the metabolic status is stabilized (otherwise they may acutely die of their metabolic problems)
What is the standard medication used to control uric acid levels in patients with tumor lysis syndrome?	Allopurinol
What newer medication is nearly always able to avert renal failure (due to uric acid levels) in tumor lysis patients?	Rasburicase (it makes the uric acid very soluble)
What is the management of last resort for acute tumor lysis patients?	Dialysis
In case you should see it on your boards, what new lab test has largely replaced "bleeding time?"	PFA – Platelet function activity
Name three ways a female could be affected by hemophilia?	• Turner syndrome (XO) • Androgen-insensitivity syndrome (XY) • Unfavorable lyonization (normal female mosaic pattern, but too many of the good Xs turned off)

A vignette is presented of a male child with a normal CBC, platelets, PT, and bleeding time. The child has a significantly elevated PTT, though. Which familial disorder is this?	**Hemophilia (Factor 8 or 9)**
Which children normally have an elevated PTT?	<6 months old
The family history of a Factor 8- or 9-deficient patient will usually be positive for _____?	**History of bleeding problems in maternal uncles**
A relatively common cause of a prolonged PTT in children, that is not due to a familial disorder, is _____?	Lupus anticoagulant (remember that lupus anticoagulant is very unfortunately named – it paradoxically causes increased clotting)
If all CBC and bleeding parameters are normal *except the bleeding time,* what kind of a disorder is it? (two possibilities)	• Aspirin effect • Platelet function disorder (hereditary)
An elevated number of megakaryocytes on bone marrow aspirates suggests what disorder?	ITP
How long must idiopathic thrombocytopenic purpura persist to call it "chronic?"	**>6 months**
What is Evans syndrome?	More than one autoimmune cytopenia, even if they occur at different times – Usually it's: ITP + immune hemolytic anemia (may be associated with later lupus in female patients)
What treatment provides the fastest response for ITP?	IVIG (very expensive, though!)
What is an important complication to be aware of, when using IVIG?	Aseptic meningitis

What age group is most likely to develop ITP in childhood?	**2–5-year-olds**
When a neonate is thrombocytopenic, what general etiology is most likely?	**Maternal causes** (mainly isoimmune or maternal ITP)
Acute ITP is more common in which gender during childhood?	Males
Chronic ITP is more common in which gender during childhood?	Females
How is the response to steroids different in acute vs. chronic ITP?	Good with acute Variable with chronic
How is the response to IVIG different in acute vs. chronic ITP?	Good with acute Short-lived for chronic
Is acute ITP more common in young children, or older children?	Young
In general, what controversy exists about treatment for DIC?	Whether to give FFP/cryoprecipitate to promote clotting (which might lead to more damaging micro-clots) Or Heparin to prevent further clotting (which might worsen bleeding but also might prevent using up more clotting factors – it's an attempt to stop the cascade)
Historically, we have waited for hemophiliacs to have bleeding problems before beginning treatment. What is the current recommendation?	Prophylactic treatment produces much better long-term function
Which is more common, deficiency of Factor 8 or 9?	Factor 8 (1 per 10,000 vs. 1 per 50,000)
If a patient has "severe" Factor 8 or 9 deficiency, what does that say about their factor activity level?	**<1 % activity!**

If a hemophiliac has a bleeding incident, what is the target factor level?	Depends: Minor – up to 30 % Moderate – up to 75 % Severe – 75 – 100 %
What sort of bleeding is considered "minor" for a hemophiliac?	Soft tissue bleeds and hematuria
What sort of bleeding is considered severe for a hemophiliac?	CNS bleeds, major trauma, surgery, retropharyngeal, or retroperitoneal bleeding
What is the characteristic appearance of hemophiliacs?	Muscle wasting, due to multiple bleeding incidents in soft tissue over time
What is the most common inherited disorder in the US Caucasian population?	von Willebrand's disease (1 %)
What over-the-counter medication should von Willebrand's patients be especially careful to avoid?	Aspirin
What are the lab parameters expected for von Willebrand's patients?	↑ PTT ↑ Bleeding time ↓ Factor 8
When von Willebrand's patients bleed, what are the main treatments?	DDAVP & vWF concentrate (Factor 8 concentrates are sometimes used, but they are only helpful if they are not very pure, and therefore still contain von Willebrand's factor)
If you have a child with a hypercoagulable disorder, what is the best therapeutic option in kids?	**Low-molecular-weight heparins**
Which are more common in kids – carcinomas or sarcomas?	**Sarcomas**
90 % of Hodgkin lymphoma patients have what finding at presentation?	**Cervical adenopathy** – painless, rubbery, & matted

Clinically localized Hodgkin disease usually turns out to be what type?	Nodular sclerotic (NS) (about 75 % of adolescent cases & 45 % of cases in younger children)
Which type of Hodgkin lymphoma is unusually common in young children (before adolescence)?	Mixed cellularity (about 33 %)
What does anemia in a Hodgkin patient indicate?	Could be either advanced disease or autoimmune hemolysis
Non-Hodgkin lymphoma patients are at special risk for what cardiac complication?	Pericardial effusion
What percentage of Burkitt lymphoma cases is related to EBV in the USA?	15 % (associated, but not super high)
A male child with lower extremity and scrotal edema could have what sort of tumor?	Something compressing the IVC – often neuroblastoma
A classic presentation of neuroblastoma involving the head and neck is?	**Raccoon eyes & proptosis**
Which paraneoplastic syndromes are common in neuroblastoma?	Opsomyoclonus (myoclonic jerks & dancing eyes) & intractable secretory diarrhea (due to VIP secretion)
If a rhabdomyosarcoma is described as "botryoid," what does that mean?	It is shaped like a bunch of polyps – often seen when this tumor develops in the GU tract
What sort of cells make a rhabdomyosarcoma?	Mesenchymal cells that were supposed to become skeletal muscle (that's why they can occur anywhere)
Wilms tumors are especially associated with what two physical exam findings?	Hemihypertrophy & aniridia

The name of the Wilms tumor precursor lesion is _____?

"Nephrogenic rests"
(also known as nephroblastomatosis)

The most common bone tumor in kids is _____?

Osteosarcoma

When and where is an osteosarcoma most likely to occur?

• Adolescence

Metaphyses of rapidly growing bones (usually on either side of the knee, or the proximal humerus)

How is osteosarcoma treated?

Excision – but limb-sparing surgery with artificial replacement of bone is now preferred

+

Chemotherapy
(80 % survival)

Which genetic mutations are associated with osteosarcoma?

RB & p53

Is it common for osteosarcoma patients to have obvious metastases at the time of presentation?

Yes – about 1 in 5 have obvious metastases

Where does osteosarcoma like to go when it metastasizes?

The lungs
(and other bone sites, of course)

Which ethnic group usually develops Ewing's sarcoma?

Caucasians
(usually in adolescence)

Are sickle cell patients at increased risk for stroke?

Yes

Should sickle cell patients be routinely screened for stroke risk?

Yes – annual transcranial Doppler (follow-up with MRA if needed)

At what age is transcranial Doppler examination for stroke risk usually discontinued?

16 years old

What is the role of transfusion therapy for patients with sickle cell, in terms of stroke risk?

Chronic transfusion therapy reduces stroke risk in patients with abnormal findings on transcranial Doppler (≥200 cm/s)

How effective is transfusion therapy in reducing the risk of stroke for patients with abnormal Doppler results?

>90 %!!!

What treatment can cure thalassemia?

Bone marrow transplant

If a patient has a family history positive for gall stones at an early age, and a few family members had splenectomies, what inherited disorder is the issue?

Spherocytosis

Fever, dark urine, and splenomegaly after travel to Nicaragua =

Malaria

8-year-old female with easy bruising, bleeding from gums, joint pain, and fever for 2 weeks =

ALL (usually)

Fever, exudative tonsillitis, hepatosplenomegaly =

EBV

Fever, bone pain, sudden movements of extremities and eyes =

Neuroblastoma (opsomyoclonus)

Cutaneous nodules in a newborn could be what two oncological problems?

Neuroblastoma

Or

Leukemia

Birbeck granules go with what malignancy?

Langerhans cell histiocytosis (LCH) (Letterer-Siwe or multisystem LCH is the most severe form and develops in kids <2 years old – presents with head, abdomen, and intertriginal rash)

A two-and-a-half-year-old white male with persistent skin rash and history of recurrent pneumonias now has platelets of only 40,000. What is the disorder?	Wiskott-Aldrich
Lytic lesion at the growth plate of the femur + positive bone scan =	**Osteosarcoma**
Regression of milestones + anemia/ thrombocytopenia with splenomegaly + cherry red spot =	**Niemann-Pick**
11-year-old white male with short stature + low white count + fatty pancreatic infiltrates =	**Shwachman-Diamond**
Most common cause of neutropenia?	**Viral illness** (second most common is normal variation due to inheritance and/or racial variation)
9-year-old white male already diagnosed with both basal and squamous cell skin cancers. Diagnosis?	Xeroderma pigmentosum
Headache + early morning vomiting + blurred vision =	Intracerebral tumor
A 13-year-old white male complains of fever, constipation, and abdominal pain. What oncology problem could be to blame?	Non-Hodgkin lymphoma
A 14-year-old white female has fever, night sweats, and all-over itching. She has a little lump in her supraclavicular area. Diagnosis?	Hodgkin lymphoma
Adolescent with a seizure disorder, mr, and malar spots that look like acne. Diagnosis?	Tuberous sclerosis

In addition to congenital disorders and trauma, why might a patient be anemic?
 	
   (3 general categories)
	1. Medication side effect
	2. Chronic disease
	   (including rheumatologic ones)
	3. Poor nutrition (vitamin/mineral deficiencies)

How do you know whether an anemia is microcytic or macrocytic?	Check the "mean corpuscular volume" (MCV) *(normal is 80–100 for adolescents, for newborns 100–120, for children it's 70s, increasing toward the adolescent level)*
The quantity of reticulocytes in the RBC sample is usually given as an index (%). What should the reticulocyte index be in an anemic patient?	>2 % (otherwise the marrow is not responding to the anemia, and it may be the problem)
The important causes of macrocytic anemia are _____? (4)	1. B12 deficiency 2. Alcoholism/liver dz 3. Reaction to drugs (phenytoin, methotrexate) 4. Folate deficiency Mnemonic: Spells BARF!
Jaundice + anemia, especially if both conjugated & unconjugated bili are high = what general diagnosis?	Hemolytic anemia
Schistocytes, "helmet" cells, microspherocytes, and RBC fragments indicate what type of anemia?	Hemolytic anemia (looks like bites have been taken out of the cells)
Basophilic stippling of RBCs in an anemic patient indicates what diagnosis?	Lead exposure
Spherocytes on the peripheral blood smear of an anemia patient indicates what two possible causes of the anemia?	1. Hereditary spherocytosis 2. Hemolytic anemia (including from incompatibility between maternal & fetal blood types)

Folate & B_{12} deficiency both produce what change in the neutrophils?	Hypersegmentation of the nucleus
Patients with splenic dysfunction develop what RBC finding?	Howell-Jolly bodies
A patient has his spleen removed after a traumatic injury. He is later noted to have little blue areas in his RBCs. What are these called, and why are they there?	• Howell-Jolly bodies • Indicates splenic dysfunction or absence (usually just one per cell)
Hypersegmented neutrophils are seen with which two types of anemia?	B_{12} & folate deficiency
Which two "mechanical" problems sometimes cause anemia?	1. Mechanical valves 2. Microangiopathic vessel changes that damage & use up RBCs
On phsyical exam, what do you expect to find with anemic patients?	1. Tachycardia 2. Pallor **3. Systolic ejection murmur**
What do anemia patients usually see the doctor for?	1. Tachypnea or palpitations 2. Fatigue 3. Dizzy/light-headed
Why do anemia patients often have systolic ejection murmurs?	High flow (same reason healthy pregnant patients often have a murmur)
What causes of microcytic anemia are important to know about?	1. Lead 2. Iron deficiency 3. Thalassemia 4. Anemia of chronic disease 5. Sideroblastic anemia Mnemonic: Spells LITAS. Put it together with the macrocytic mnemonic, and you have "LITAS BARF"

What is the most common cause of anemia in the USA?	Iron deficiency (typically seen in young, menstruating females and toddlers with poor dietary intake and/or excessive milk consumption)
What odd behavior sometimes occurs along with anemia?	Craving for ice, dirt, and other non-nutritive substances (Called "pica")
How is iron-deficiency anemia treated?	1. Treat with iron 2. Search for the cause & correct it
If iron-deficiency anemia occurs in a patient who is not menstruating, what is the likely cause?	Occult GI bleeding
What is Plummer-Vinson syndrome?	1. Esophageal webbing 2. Iron-deficiency anemia 3. Glossitis (tongue inflammation)
In what patient group are you most likely to see Plummer-Vinson syndrome?	Women of northern European & British ancestry
Anemia + a skull X-ray with a "crew-cut" appearance is what disorder?	Thalassemia (occasionally sickle cell)
If a patient has G6PD deficiency, what would you expect to see on the blood smear?	Heinz bodies

Mnemonic: Think of them as Heinz 57 varieties – because so many things induce G6PD! |
| If anemia has a bone marrow cause, what are the three usual reasons to think of? | 1. Aplastic anemia (lack of all cell types) 2. Myelofibrotic/myelophthisic changes (marrow replaced by fibrous stuff) 3. Sideroblastic anemia (various problems forming Hgb lead to sideroblastic anemia) |
| How can you identify the cells of sideroblastic anemia? | 1. They are in the marrow (usually) 2. They have iron-inclusion bodies in the RBC |

If the peripheral blood smear report says "polychromasia," what should you conclude?

There are probably immature blood cells circulating
(possible hemolytic anemia)

Echinocytes or "burr cells" mean that what condition is affecting your patient?

Uremia!

Myelofibrosis causes what unusual RBC shape?

Tear-drop-shaped RBCs
(and anemia)

Microangiopathic diseases cause what kind of RBC changes?

Chewed up cells –
Helmets, schistocytes, & fragments

Echinocytes ("prickly-looking" cells), or "burr cells," go with what metabolic problem?

Uremia

Target cells go with which diseases?

1. Thalassemia
2. Liver disease

If many new RBCs are being made, what will their appearance be on micro exam?

Polychromasia
(part blue, part red – due to immaturity)

Parasites inside the RBCs should make you think of which two diagnoses?

1. Malaria
2. Babesiosis (often contracted at the same time as Lyme disease)

Lead poisoning causes what typical RBC change?

Basophilic stippling
(tiny blue dots)

Uremia produces what characteristic change in the RBCs?

Burr cells
(aka echinocytes – due to their prickly appearance)

Tear-drop-shaped RBCs often occur in what disease process?

Myelofibrosis

G6PD deficiency produces a special RBC appearance. What is it?

The Heinz body

What does a Heinz body look like?

Small, round, blue inclusions in the RBC

Are Heinz bodies bad for the RBC?	Yes – They cause the damage that leads to hemolysis
Why are "bite cells" sometimes seen in G6PD?	Splenic macrophages "bit out" the Heinz body *(this may not be the actual mechanism, but it is a useful way to remember it – Heinz™ makes a lot of tasty products, after all!)*
Why can small numbers of spherocytes sometimes be seen in hemolytic anemias?	RBCs with abnormally small surface areas sometimes end up round
Why does G6PD seldom produce a dangerous anemia?	Only older RBCs are affected (young RBCs are able to synthesize new enzyme, if some is damaged)
How is G6PD inherited?	X-linked! (recessive)
Which patients are most likely to have G6PD deficiency?	• African-Americans & Mediterraneans • Men (X-linked) (It's prevalent in malarious areas, just like sickle cell is)
What is the problem with G6PD deficiency?	RBCs lyse suddenly
How is G6PD triggered?	Only by "inducers" – Such as sulfa, salicylates, antimalarials, fava beans
Sideroblastic anemia can be identified easily if what cells are present?	RBCs in bone marrow laced with iron inclusions
Liver diseases produce what characteristic RBC change?	Target cells (also seen in thalassemia)
Myelofibrosis (aka myelophthisic change) in the bone marrow produces what unusual RBC shape?	Tear drops (The RBCs are trying to fit through the fibrous material, and it stretches out their "tails")

Microspherocytes in a newborn usually indicate what problem?

Blood type incompatibilities between mother & fetus (but can be any type of immune hemolytic anemia)

Regular spherocytes are seen in which type of disorders?

1. Hereditary spherocytosis
2. Hemolysis (occasionally)
   (microspherocytes are more common with hemolysis)

How can you know that spherocytes are due to the hereditary disorder?

The osmotic fragility test is positive (The RBC breaks easily at high osmotic pressures)

What does sideroblastic anemia indicate?

Patient is likely to develop a blood dyscrasia in the future

What is anisocytosis?

Cells are of different sizes (not "iso," which means "the same")

What is poikilocytosis?

Cells are of different shapes

Bleeding time tells you how well the _____ is working?

Platelet system

Hemophilia is a recessive disease. What dominant disorder causes increased bleeding?

von Willebrand's

Lupus has an "anticoagulant factor." Does that mean that lupus patients have difficulty clotting?

No –
They are often *hyper*coagulable

In DIC, what coagulation labs do you expect will be prolonged?

All of them
(PT/PTT & bleeding time)

Positive "split products" or "fibrin products" indicates what process is going on?

Large amounts of clotting (as in DIC or a DVT/PE)

Recurrent miscarriages & a positive VDRL test indicate what disorder?

Lupus
(The VDRL cross-reacts)

What unusual cause of platelet disorder does the board exam like to test?

Vitamin C deficiency (aka scurvy)

If a patient suddenly starts bleeding from existing puncture sites (e.g., the IV site), what does the patient have?	DIC
Sudden DIC in a young patient is seen in what three settings?	1. Trauma/fractures – fat embolism 2. Amniotic fluid embolism 3. Sepsis
Pancytopenia h/o radiation therapy Down's syndrome Child (usually age 3–5) These buzzwords = what diagnosis?	Acute lymphocytic/lymphoblastic leukemia (ALL)
What problems (symptoms) are associated with pancytopenia?	Fever Bleeding Anemia (also fatigue, pallor, & heart murmur)
What is the typical age for Hodgkin lymphoma? **(night sweats, cervical LAD)**	**15–34 years**
Which virus causes Burkitt lymphoma?	**EBV**
Where is endemic Burkitt lymphoma seen?	Africa
How does endemic Burkitt lymphoma typically present?	Jaw mass – child – African
Reed-Sternberg cell Cervical lymphadenopathy Night sweats 15–34-year-old patient These buzzwords = what diagnosis?	Hodgkin lymphoma
What causes T cell leukemia?	Unknown in children (linked to HTLV-1 in adults, but not in children)
Is T cell leukemia a significant cause of childhood ALL?	Yes – about 15 %

What patient presentation is especially suggestive of a T cell cause for ALL?

Respiratory distress and/or stridor – Due to mediastinal mass

A "dry tap" on attempted bone marrow biopsy suggests what process in a cancer patient?
(associated with CML and multiple myeloma)

Myelodysplasia/myelofibrosis aka "myelophthisic" changes

Philadelphia chromosome
Blast crisis
Splenomegaly
WBC >50,000
These buzzwords go with what diagnosis?

CML
(Chronic myelogenous leukemia – more common in adults, but also seen in children)

What types of problems accompany primary thrombocythemia?

Either bleeding or thrombosis

Reed-Sternberg cells are usually described as looking like _____?

Owl eyes

Reed-Sternberg cells are characteristic of which disorder?

Hodgkin lymphoma

"Starry sky" pattern on histology goes with what (general) type of diagnosis?

High-grade lymphoma

What is the other name for Burkitt lymphoma?
(It uses a histologic description)

Small, non-cleaved lymphoma

Overall, what are the most common general cancer types in children?

Leukemia & CNS tumors

Overall, what are the most common cancers in young adults <30 years old?
    (two general types)

Leukemia & lymphoma

If you suspect spinal cord compromise (a complication of cancer masses or sometimes of fractures due to lytic lesions), what do you do?
(4 steps)

1. Start high-dose steroids
2. Order an emergent MRI (done even at 2 a.m.!)
3. Set patient up for radiation therapy
4. Neurosurgery consult for possible surgical decompression

When is surgical decompression of a tumor needed?
(2 reasons)

1. Tumor is known to be radiation insensitive
2. Tumor fails radiation treatment when attempted

Genetic conditions associated with cancers are generally autosomal dominant except what three disorders?

1. Albinism (recessive)
2. Xeroderma pigmentosa (recessive)
3. Down syndrome (trisomy)

Ideally, where should you place an IV line in a patient with superior vena cava syndrome?

The lower extremities
(hopefully, this fluid will return to the heart unimpeded through the IVC)

What is the biggest known *modifiable* risk factor for cancer in the US population?

Smoking

If you need to biopsy a lung mass, what are your choices for how to accomplish this? Rank them from least invasive to most invasive.

1. Bronchoscopic biopsy
2. CT-guided biopsy
3. Open lung biopsy

Skin changes associated with a breast mass or nodule suggest what diagnosis?

Cancer

If a breast mass is freely mobile, does it suggest cancer or a benign diagnosis?

Benign

What are the typical findings for Horner's syndrome?

Ptosis, miosis, anhidrosis

What is a mesothelioma?

A malignant tumor of the pleura

What three environmental exposures are risk factors for later development of bladder cancer?

1. Smoking
2. Schistosomiasis
3. Aniline dye (rubber & dye industry)

What three environmental exposures are linked to the later development of liver cancers?	1. Alcohol 2. Aflatoxins (moldy peanuts) 3. Vinyl chloride (liver angiosarcomas)
What food exposure is linked to the development of stomach cancer?	Smoked meat & fish (nitrosamines & nitrites)
Clear cell cancer of the cervix or vagina is linked to what exposure?	*Maternal* DES exposure during pregnancy
What are the three main risk factors for development of cervical cancer?	1. Smoking 2. Large number of sexual partners 3. High parity
What are the commonly tested paraneoplastic syndromes associated with cancers?	1. Cushing's syndrome 2. SIADH 3. Hypercalcemia 4. Eaton-Lambert
What is Eaton-Lambert syndrome?	Myasthenia gravis-like paraneoplastic syndrome – rare in children, but occurs as an autoimmune disorder or with malignancy
How can Eaton-Lambert syndrome be differentiated from myasthenia gravis?	Repetitive use of muscles makes them *stronger* in Eaton-Lambert
Are mammograms useful in women <35 years old?	Not usually – The breast tissue is too dense
If you find a suspicious breast mass, should you get a mammogram before biopsying it?	No – Biopsy is indicated regardless of mammogram findings
With a known breast mass, how can mammography sometimes still be helpful?	May indicate other suspicious areas to investigate
What is Trousseau syndrome?	Migratory thrombophlebitis (They are really thromboemboli, but are commonly referred to as "thrombophlebitis")

Trousseau syndrome is rare in children. What is it associated with, in children?	Infection & trauma (in adults it is most often associated with neoplasms)
How can you differentiate insulinoma from factitious disorder or an accidental overdose?	C-peptide – It's high in insulinoma
How are insulinomas treated?	Resection
Are insulinomas generally benign or malignant?	Benign (90 %)
In addition to insulinomas, there are two other islet cell tumor types – what are they?	1. Glucagonoma (alpha cells) 2. VIPoma
What are the symptoms of VIPoma or VIP paraneoplastic syndrome? (3)	Mainly . . . 1. Watery diarrhea 2. Hypokalemia 3. Achlorhydria (low stomach acid)
What are the symptoms or signs of glucagonoma? (3)	1. Hyperglycemia 2. High glucagon 3. Migratory necrotizing skin erythema!
If you find a patient with an islet cell tumor, what syndrome should you look for?	MEN (Multiple endocrine neoplasia)
Describe Zollinger-Ellison syndrome.	Gastrinoma produces abnormally high gastrin levels → acid hypersecretion & bad peptic ulcer disease
In a vignette, what would suggest gastrinoma as a diagnosis? (3)	1. Multiple peptic ulcers 2. Ulcers not responsive to treatment 3. Distal intestinal ulcers
Are gastrinomas usually benign or malignant?	50/50 (Trick question)
If a stomach ulcer does not heal properly, despite appropriate medical treatment, what should you consider?	Malignancy (much more common in gastric ulcers than other types)

What is Meigs syndrome?	A benign ovarian tumor (usually fibroma) that causes ascites & right-sided hydrothorax
What common medication reduces the risk of ovarian cancer?	Oral contraceptives
Ovarian teratomas are also known by what other name?	Dermoids or dermoid cysts
Why do dermoids often show up on X-ray?	They often contain teeth or other calcifications
What are the symptoms of a Sertoli-Leydig tumor?	Boy stuff (deep voice, hairy face, receding hairline, etc.)
What are the symptoms of granulosa/ theca-cell tumors?	Feminization & precocious puberty
In general terms, what is the early sign of possible cervical cancer development?	Cervical dysplasia (on Pap smear) (prevention is now attempted through HPV vaccination, of course)
How is DES exposure related to cancer development?	Maternal DES exposure during pregnancy → clear cell cancer of the vagina or cervix
When should routine Pap smear evaluation be instituted?	When the patient is 21 years old (regardless of the age at which she becomes sexually active) *This is a change from previous practice!*
Which patients may require more frequent Pap smear monitoring, or to be monitored at younger ages?	• Those with in utero DES exposure • Immunocompromised or HIV+ • History of cervical cancer or precancer
If you have the option to get a Pap smear (on the boards) for a young woman who is due for one, what should you do?	If there are acute matters to be managed, choose an answer related to the acute problems – If not, get it even if the presenting complaint is unrelated

How should dysplastic Pap smear results be followed up in a young, healthy female? | Repeat in 6–12 months

If a young woman requires Pap smear evaluation, should HPV DNA testing also be done? | No –
HPV DNA+ findings are common & often transient in this group, so testing is not recommended

Which HPV types are most associated with the development of cervical cancer? | Types 16 & 18

Which HPV types are included in the quadrivalent HPV vaccine? | 16 & 18
(most linked to cervical cancer)
6 & 11
(most linked to anogenital warts)

If there is persistent dysplasia on the Pap smear for a young woman, how do you complete their evaluation? (multi-step) | 1. Colposcopy
2. Directed biopsy
3. Endocervical sampling

What are the main risk factors for cervical cancer?
(5 – three are behavioral) | 1. Age <20 first coitus
2. Multiple sexual partners/promiscuous partner
3. Smoking
4. Low socioeconomic status (SES)
5. High parity

Elevated AFP is associated with which two cancers? | 1. Liver
2. TESTICULAR!

The S-100 marker is associated with what general types of tumors?
(3) | CNS, nerve, and melanoma tumors
(Remember that melanocytes are closely related to CNS cells)

HCG will be elevated in non-pregnant women with what two disorders? | 1. Hydatidiform mole
2. Choriocarcinoma

If a child presents with bilateral retinoblastoma, what does that tell you about the nature of the disorder? | It is the inherited form

If you should see intracranial calcifications on a skull X-ray, what tumor diagnosis is suggested?

Craniopharyngioma
(or meningioma, if it's at the edge of the skull, but they are rare in kids)

Signs of 7th & 8th cranial nerve damage could be due to which tumor?

Acoustic neuroma

What tumor is usually described as looking like a "bunch of grapes," and is seen in children?

Sarcoma botryoides
(a vaginal tumor – it's a subtype of rhabdomyosarcoma!)

Why does polycystic ovary syndrome increase the risk of endometrial cancer?

It causes unopposed estrogen stimulation (chronically)

In general, what two processes increase the risk for endometrial cancer?

1. Chronic elevation of estrogen
2. Increased number of proliferative cycles

How are brain tumors treated, in general?

Resection, if possible –
Then radiation and/or chemo depending on tumor type

What is the most common solid malignancy in adult men <30 years old?

Testicular cancer

What is the main risk factor for testicular cancer?

Cryptorchidism

What risk factor is known to increase the chance of testicular cancer in childhood, before adolescence?

Intersex conditions with ambiguous genitalia

How can ultrasound, or simple transillumination, help you distinguish testicular cancer from other masses?

Cancer is *not* fluid filled
(and will not transilluminate)

If you are concerned about a possible testicular cancer, how do you diagnose it?
    (3 steps)

1. Ultrasound (to better define the structures present – normal and abnormal)
2. AFP & HCG tumor marker labs
3. Surgical examination & biopsy

What is the most common type of testicular cancer, overall?

Seminoma

Before puberty, how common are testicular seminomas?	Rare
Which tumors are the most common testicular tumors for prepubertal boys?	Yolk sac tumors & Teratomas (80 % of prepubertal tumors are one of these types)
About 10 % of the testicular tumors seen in prepubertal boys come from which general tumor group?	Gonadal stromal tumors (meaning Sertoli cell, Leydig cell, or juvenile granulosa cell tumors – Sertoli cell is most common)
If AFP is elevated in a patient with a testicular tumor, which tumor types does that suggest? (2)	Yolk sac Or Embryonal carcinoma
How are testicular cancers treated?	Resection, followed by radiation, chemotherapy, or observation, depending on type
What is the prognosis for patients with a seminoma?	Excellent (a tumor generally not seen before adolescence)
Which prepubertal testicular tumors are benign, and only require resection to cure them?	Sertoli cell tumors Leydig cell tumors & teratomas
Leukocoria and exophthalmos suggest what diagnosis?	Retinoblastoma
What is leukocoria?	A *white,* rather than red, pupillary light reflex
These buzzwords = what diagnosis? Headache Papilledema Vomiting Obese young woman Normal head CT	Pseudotumor cerebri

Which ethnic population is most likely to develop nasopharyngeal cancer?	Asians
Which virus is associated with nasopharyngeal cancer development?	EBV
How is liver cancer treated, in general?	Surgery and chemotherapy
What is the most common type of pituitary tumor?	Craniopharyngioma (in children) *(Prolactinoma is more common for older patients)*
What is the classic finding with pituitary tumors?	Bitemporal hemianopsia
What additional symptoms might a person with a prolactinoma develop? (4)	1. Galactorrhea 2. Menstrual dysfunction 3. Sexual dysfunction 4. Signs of elevated ICP
Is a liver hemangioma benign or malignant?	Benign (no treatment needed unless symptomatic)
Which patients develop hepatic adenomas?	Young women on oral contraceptives
How are hepatic adenomas treated in that population?	Discontinue the oral contraceptives (it will regress or stop growing)
Hepatoblastoma is the most common primary liver tumor for what group of patients?	Children
Increased calcitonin in a patient with a thyroid mass suggests what problem?	Medullary thyroid cancer (usually MEN related)
Describe the typical thyroid cancer mass.	Single, hard, non-tender, & "cold" on scan
A thyroid cancer patient who develops hoarseness probably has what problem?	Involvement of the recurrent laryngeal nerve

What environmental exposure, formerly used as a medical treatment, is linked to the later development of thyroid cancer?

Neck irradiation (previously used to treat hyperthyroidism – sometimes also used as a treatment for acne)

What is the best way to evaluate a thyroid nodule?

Fine-needle aspiration

Or

Open biopsy if very suspicious

What are the least invasive ways to do a preliminary thyroid nodule evaluation?
(3)

1. Check TSH/TFTs
2. Nuclear scan
3. Ultrasound (if it's a cyst, it's probably benign)

What is the other name for Conn syndrome?

Primary hyperaldosteronism

How should you evaluate any skin lesion you suspect could be cancer?

Biopsy

What is the main risk factor for skin cancers of the squamous or basal cell type?

UV light exposure

Where are osteosarcomas usually found?

About the knee (femur or tibia)

At what age do people develop osteosarcomas, generally?

Between 10 & 30 years

How is an osteosarcoma supposed to look on X-ray?

Like a "sunburst"

Which bones are at greatest risk for later development of osteosarcoma?
(2)

1. Tibia or femur
2. Those that have had a high rate of turnover (h/o osteomyelitis, for example, but this factor is seen more often in adult osteosarcoma than in childhood cases)

What are the typical symptoms of a carcinoid (neuroendocrine) tumor?

1. Flushing
2. Diarrhea
3. Abdominal cramping
4. Heart valve damage

What determines when a carcinoid tumor becomes symptomatic?

When it metastasizes *to the liver*

(Before the tumor reaches the liver, the products it makes are destroyed by the liver, so symptoms are rare)

What is the main molecule secreted by carcinoid tumors?

Serotonin

What serum level is elevated (reliably) in carcinoid tumor patients?

5-Hydroxy-indole-acetic acid (a serotonin product)

In general terms, where does carcinoid usually originate?

Small bowel

What is the most common tumor of the appendix?

Carcinoid

What is the most common GI tract tumor in children?

Carcinoid

Primary pulmonary tumors are rare in children. When they do occur, what is the most common tumor type?

Carcinoid (also known as a neuroendocrine tumor, or NET)

How do you decide whether a spot on the skin is suspicious for melanoma?

Asymmetry
Borders (irregular – bad)
Color (multiple or change)
Diameter (bigger is worse)

What is the main predictor of whether a melanoma will metastasize?

Depth of skin invasion

(but they often metastasize very early, regardless of depth)

How should a suspected melanoma be evaluated?

Excisional biopsy

(You would prefer to get all of it out, if possible)

For patients with advanced or unresectable melanoma, what general category of treatments has been recently approved?

Immunotherapies

(usually targeting PD-1 or PD-L1 proteins that tumors use to "turn off" the cytotoxic immune response)

A pearly, telangiectatic lesion, often with a raised border, suggests what diagnosis?	Basal cell cancer (rare in children, but sometimes seen, most often on the head)
How should you evaluate a pearly, telangiectatic skin lesion?	Excisional biopsy
Prevention is an important aspect of pediatric care, especially in adolescence. What are the main behavioral risk factors to consider for later development of oral cancers?	1. ETOH 2. Smoking 3. Chewing tobacco
What is the initial appearance of oral cancer (usually)?	Leukoplakia
Is "oral hairy leukoplakia" the same thing as "leukoplakia?"	No – Plain leukoplakia is an early oral cancer ("oral hairy leukoplakia is an AIDS-related disease associated with EBV)
Are "unicameral bone cysts" benign or malignant?	**Benign**
Which patient population tends to develop unicameral bone cysts?	**Children & adolescents**
How can a unicameral bone cyst cause problems?	**If large enough, pathological fractures can occur**
These buzzwords = what diagnosis? Expansile lesion of proximal Humerus Lytic lesion Patient <18 years old	**Unicameral bone cyst** (benign)
If an expansile cystic bone lesion expands beyond the diameter of the bone, what is the likely diagnosis?	Osteosarcoma

Wilms tumor & neuroblastoma can be difficult to differentiate. What is one radiographic way to tell them apart?	*Wilms tumor* is a *kidney* tumor, so the calyceal architecture is often disrupted by it – *Neuroblastoma should not affect renal architecture* (it is usually coming from the adrenal)
Why do anemic patients sometimes have systolic ejection murmurs?	**Because they have high flow (high cardiac output) due to the low hemoglobin content of the blood**
Hypersegmented neutrophils in an anemic patient = what diagnosis?	**Folate or B$_{12}$ deficiency (macrocytic)**
If the peripheral blood smear shows "polychromasia," what underlying process is probably going on?	**Reticulocytosis (usually due to hemolysis)**
Why do some antibiotics cause anemia?	PCNs and cephalosporins can cause RBC antibody formation → hemolysis
What life-threatening complication of cancer produces hypotension, JVD, and narrow pulse pressure?	**Pericardial effusion**
In addition to the cancer, itself, why else might cancer patients develop tamponade?	**As a complication of radiation or chemotherapy**
What determines how acutely ill a patient with tamponade will be? (2)	1. Amount of fluid 2. How fast it accumulates
How does the chest X-ray for a patient with tamponade look?	Depends . . . Slow accumulation → cardiomegaly without CHF Rapid accumulation → normal or near-normal appearance
What is the treatment for SVC syndrome?	**Radiation therapy (RT)**

How can you treat an SVC patient until RT is available?

Diuretics

&

Steroids
(temporary measures only)

What is an acceptable alternative to MRI to evaluate for spinal cord compression?

CT myelography X-ray

(contrast is injected into the CSF space)

In a cancer patient, new onset of urinary retention should suggest what problem?

Possible spinal cord compression

(also consider medications & urological causes)

What skin cancer has a special interest in causing pericardial effusions?

Malignant melanoma

How is pericardial effusion treated acutely?

Pericardiocentesis/
pericardial window
(a surgical procedure to permit ongoing evaluation & drainage)

How is pericardial effusion caused by cancer metastases treated for the long term?

Intrapericardial chemo

Or

Radiation therapy

How can you treat a hyperviscosity syndrome in an oncology patient?
(3)

1. Hydration
2. Phlebotomy
3. Plasmapheresis

When does your oncology patient with SIADH require more aggressive treatment than fluid restriction?

With seizures or cardiac arrhythmia
(give hypertonic saline)

How much hydrocortisone would you give a pediatric oncology patient who is hypotensive – with suspected adrenal insufficiency?

50–75 mg/m^2 initially, followed by the same dose divided into four IV doses given over time

Why is hydrocortisone preferred in a hypotensive, hyponatremic, or hyperkalemic patient with adrenal insufficiency?

Hydrocortisone has mineralocorticoid effects, which these patients need

Which steroid replacement form is preferred for patients in whom adrenal insufficiency is suspected, but not certain? Why?

Dexamethasone –
It does not interfere with the cosyntropin stimulation test, used to evaluate for adrenal insufficiency

(Hydrocortisone will affect the results of this test)

What is the second most common (general) type of cancer in children?

**CNS tumors
(leukemias are #1)**

What is the typical location for a childhood primary CNS tumor?

Cerebellum or posterior fossa

(2/3 of all childhood CNS tumors are infratentorial)

What is the typical location for an adult-onset primary CNS tumor?

Supratentorial (2/3)

**Mnemonic:
Adults are taller, so their tumors are higher!**

Which children are most likely to develop ALL?

**Boys
Age 3–5
White
Industrialized nation**

Stridor, orthopnea, or shortness of breath in an ALL patient suggests what problem?

Mediastinal mass

Bone pain, limping, and arthralgia in an ALL patient suggest what problem?

Infiltrative disease of the marrow

Sternal tenderness in an ALL patient suggests what diagnosis?

Marrow infiltration

Bleeding in the eyes, mucosa, or skin of an ALL patient suggests what complication?	Thrombocytopenia Or Coagulopathy
Should a hospitalized ALL patient be isolated from other children?	No – But they should be isolated from ill children, and those with varicella (isolation is needed if the patient is post-bone marrow transplant, though, and in some cases if neutropenia develops following chemotherapy)
Are siblings of an ALL patient at higher risk for ALL?	Yes – 20 % concordance for monozygotic twins (2–4x increase in regular siblings)
Oliguria in an ALL patient suggests what problem?	Renal failure/insufficiency
Why do ALL patients develop hepato-splenomegaly?	Infiltration of those organs by leukemic cells
Testicular enlargement in a boy with ALL suggests what problem?	Testicular infiltration
Swelling of the face (and sometimes orthopnea) suggests what ALL complication?	Superior vena cava syndrome
Dependent edema and shortness of breath in an ALL patient suggest what complication?	Congestive heart failure (due to severe anemia)
The WBC count is generally above what level in ALL?	10,000 (although it's often lower)
What percentage of children with ALL has a mediastinal mass at the time of diagnosis?	5–10 %

What is the best way to screen for a mediastinal mass in children?	Screening CXR
How common are anemia & thrombocytopenia in ALL patients?	Very common – *80 % are anemic* *75 % are thrombocytopenic!*
What is the main test used to diagnose ALL?	Bone marrow aspirate >25% leukemic lymphoblasts=ALL
In a cancer patient, what do these labs suggest? **Increased LDH** **Increased uric acid** **Increased phosphate** **Increased potassium** **Low calcium**	Tumor lysis syndrome
What is the probability of getting remission for ALL?	95 % (long-term survival 80–85 % at 5 years)
Can ALL kids receive vaccinations, while they are in treatment?	No – except for the inactivated flu vaccine (Family & household members – no live vaccines during treatment)
There are six characteristics that make ALL "high risk." What are they?	1. Age <1 year or >10 years 2. WBCs >50,000 3. Bulky masses (including mediastinal masses) 4. Certain translocations (MLL & Philadelphia chromosome) 5. T cell or mature B cell disease 6. Hypoploidy (<46 chromosomes in affected cell line)
If a patient has CNS leukemia, what are the treatment options? **(2)**	Cranial radiation & Intrathecal chemotherapy (methotrexate/cytarabine/ hydrocortisone)

Do all CNS leukemia patients require treatment with both modalities?

No –
Some can receive intrathecal chemotherapy only

What are the main complications of the treatment for CNS leukemia?

1. **Growth retardation**
2. **Secondary tumors**
3. **Decline of intellectual function**

What are the four phases of ALL treatment?

1. **Induction**
2. **Consolidation**
3. **Delayed intensification**
4. **Maintenance**

Mnemonic:
It's like student loans – First you get them (induction). Then, you graduate and consolidate them. Next, you start working and "intensify" your attempt to pay them back. Finally, you get tired and switch to a steady level of payments, the "maintenance phase"

Which drugs usually used in ALL induction?
(3 regular chemo agents; 1 intrathecal group)

1. **Prednisone**
2. **Vincristine**
3. **L-Asparaginase**
4. **Intrathecal methotrexate/cytarabine/ hydrocortisone**
(+/– doxorubicin)

Mnemonic:
ALL patients need to eat their *asparagus* to increase *VIM* and *preddiness (prettiness = prednisone) (VIM = VIncristine & Intrathecal Methotrexate)*

What are three important complications of prednisone use?
(3)

1. **Cushingoid habitus**
2. **Avascular necrosis of bone**
3. **Hypertension**

What are the main complications of L-asparaginase use?
(2)

1. **Pancreatitis**
2. **Coagulopathy (often leading to cerebral infarcts)**

Mnemonic: Think of asparagus getting stuck in the pancreas and also plugging up CNS vessels

What is the main complication of doxorubicin?	**Cardiotoxicity!**
What is methotrexate's main systemic toxicity?	**Hepatotoxic**
Vincristine is responsible for the hair loss of ALL treatment. What two other complications does this medication cause?	**1. Peripheral neuropathies (reversible) – including foot drop & effects on the gut, causing constipation!** **2. SIADH**
During induction, what special support is given to the renal system?	**Aggressive hydration**
How should the CNS be protected in high-risk ALL patients without CNS involvement at diagnosis?	**Triple intrathecal chemo meds** **+** **Cranial radiation (done during consolidation phase in some high-risk patients)**
Which patients with suspected leukemia or lymphoma are usually admitted? (3 criteria)	**1. Blasts on peripheral smear** **2. Pancytopenia (or very serious thrombocytopenia <30K)** **3. Those with lymph nodes needing biopsy (may also be done outpatient)**
How does Hodgkin disease most often present in children?	**Firm, nontender nodules (LAD) in the chest or neck** **+** **Systemic symptoms (fever, night sweats, cough, & weight loss)**
What are the three most common reasons for supraclavicular lymphadenopathy?	**1. Infection** **2. Neoplasm** **3. Sarcoid (not very common in children)**
What section of the body do the supraclavicular lymph nodes drain?	**Lungs, abdomen, & mediastinum** *(not neck!)*

Is leukemic infiltration of testes or ovaries painful?	No – It is *painless* enlargement
"Hypothalamic syndrome" is an unusual CNS manifestation of leukemia. What is it?	Marked hyperphagia Weight gain Personality changes *(due to infiltration/damage to the hypothalamus)*
The symptoms of acute lymphoblastic leukemia are usually due to what secondary problem?	The decrease in normal hematopoietic elements (RBCs, WBCs, & pltlts)
What malignancy sometimes presents as an apparent peritonsillar abscess?	Primary non-Hodgkin lymphoma tumors of Waldeyer's ring (Waldeyer's ring is at the back of the mouth)
If a lymphoma patient develops abdominal pain or symptoms of obstruction, what diagnoses should be ruled out?	1. Intussusception (the tumor may serve as a lead point) 2. Small bowel obstruction (due to a developing tumor)
How does Burkitt lymphoma present when it is seen in the US?	Retroperitoneal or mesenteric tumors, and occasionally maxillary sinus tumors
Name a childhood malignancy other than leukemia that sometimes replaces the marrow?	Neuroblastoma
How can it be distinguished from leukemia based on a simple blood test?	No blast forms are seen in the peripheral blood
How can pertussis sometimes mimic leukemia in terms of lab results?	Pertussis sometimes causes a big time leukocytosis (>100,000) with neutropenia
How do storage disorders (such as Gaucher's) sometimes mimic leukemia?	They cause hepatosplenomegaly & sometimes pancytopenia

The most common mimics of leukemia/lymphoma in children are what three infectious diseases?	1. Epstein-Barr virus infection 2. Cytomegalovirus 3. Toxoplasmosis
At what ANC level are patients at risk for gram-negative infections? (ANC = absolute neutrophil count)	<500
If a neutropenic patient has pneumonia, what unusual pathogens should you worry about?	Opportunistic ones + those that are more common in hospitalized patients (Pneumocystis, Aspergillus, Legionella, Listeria)
Indwelling IV catheters put patients at special risk for what two infections?	Bacteremia & Endocarditis (usually due to staph or strep)
Mucositis in a neutropenic patient puts that patient at risk for what dangerous GI problem?	Intestinal perforation
In a neutropenic patient with intestinal perforation, what must you remember about the presentation?	Symptoms may be very mild due to limited immune response
A febrile neutropenic patient with an indwelling catheter needs what antibiotic?	Third-generation cephalosporins or equivalent medications – Cefepime, piperacillin-tazobactam, meropenem, or imipenem-cilastatin (& other categories for resistance, complications, etc.)
What meds should febrile neutropenic patients receive, in general?	The same ones
An asymptomatic neutropenic patient should generally be on what prophylactic medication, to protect against PCP infection?	TMP/SMX

If a neutropenic patient presents with pneumonia, what special antibiotic might you want to add?	TMP/SMX at treatment dose (to cover PCP)
How do you treat severe hyperkalemia in a cancer patient?	Just like any other patient: Calcium, glucose, insulin, & bicarb, then Kayexalate® (dialysis can also be used)
When can kayexalate, alone, be used to treat hyperkalemia?	Mild hyperkalemia *without EKG changes* (can be given orally or rectally)
If you suspect intestinal perforation, what antibiotic would you add to the regular febrile neutropenic medications?	Metronidazole or clindamycin (cover anaerobes)
What is the most common cause of splenomegaly in kids?	Benign viral infection
What problems does splenomegaly cause? (4)	1. Anemia (sequestration) 2. Neutropenia 3. Thrombocytopenia 4. Risk of rupture!
What are the typical causes of splenomegaly? (4)	1. Infectious disease 2. Congestion due to outflow obstruction 3. Storage diseases (e.g., Gaucher's) 4. Trauma
If you encounter an enlarged spleen in an otherwise well child, what should you do?	Nothing – Recheck in 2 months or consider checking a CBC
What criteria mean that you need to evaluate splenomegaly further? (3)	1. Still present after 2 months 2. Extends to >2 cm below the ribs 3. Associated symptoms present
What five types of crises are seen with sickle cell disease?	1. Vasoocclusive (pain crisis) 2. Aplastic 3. Sequestration 4. Hemolytic 5. Acute chest syndrome

How long do aplastic crises usually last?	**7–10 days**
What is the typical trigger for an aplastic crisis, in general terms?	**Viruses** *(especially Parvovirus B19)*
Is AML more likely to affect girls or boys?	**Affects both equally**
If a leukemia develops in the first 4 weeks of life, what type is it likely to be?	**AML** (Acute myeloid leukemia)
What is the prognosis for AML in children?	**>50 % are surviving 5 years later**
How successful is intensive chemotherapy for AML?	**85 % achieve remission**
On cytology, how are the cells of ALL and AML different?	**ALL cells are PAS+** **AML cells are PAS–** (**AML cells are positive for Sudan black & myeloperoxidase, though**)
How are the presentations of ALL and AML different?	**In general, they're the same**
How is AML diagnosed, officially?	**>20 % blasts on bone marrow aspirate**
What antifungal medications are sometimes used as prophylaxis in AML? (2)	**Fluconazole** & **Nystatin**
What two types of medications are definitely used in treating (inducing) AML?	**Anthracyclines (daunorubicin)** & **ARA-C**
Why should you avoid using blood products from patient family members when treating leukemia patients?	**Allogeneic transplant may be needed later – you don't want to "prime" the immune system against these cells**

What percentage of neuroblastoma tumors occurs <u>above</u> the diaphragm?	20 %
What percentage of neuroblastoma tumors develop from the adrenal gland?	50 %
In what age group do you usually see neuroblastoma?	**<4 years** **(1/7,000 live births)**
Do most children presenting with neuroblastoma have solitary tumors or disseminated disease?	**Disseminated**
Neuroblastoma metastasizes to what sites, in general? (5)	1. Liver 2. Bone 3. Bone marrow 4. Lymph nodes 5. Skin
Bluish nodules are noted in the skin of a neuroblastoma patient. The nodules are non-tender. What are they?	**Skin metastases** (one version of "blueberry muffin baby")
What three paraneoplastic syndromes are neuroblastoma patients likely to develop?	1. VIP syndrome 2. Catecholamine excess 3. Opsoclonus-myoclonus
What is "opsoclonus-myoclonus syndrome?"	**Dancing eyes & dancing feet (myoclonus) with or without cerebellar ataxia** *(associated with neuroblastoma, remember!)*
How is opsoclonus-myoclonus syndrome treated?	**Steroids, IVIG, & tumor treatment – Does not always resolve**
What are the three bad prognostics for neuroblastoma?	1. Age >1 year 2. Metastatic disease 3. N-myc gene amplification

Why do sickle cell patients sometimes present with RUQ pain & jaundice?	Chronic hemolysis leads to gall stone formation – obstruction produces colic
Sickle cell crisis is most commonly the result of what process?	Vasoocclusive events (due to sludging of sickled RBCs)
What is the most common presentation of vasoocclusive sickle cell crisis in children <2 years old?	Dactylitis (aka "hand-foot" syndrome)
What CNS problems are seen in children with sickle cell disease?	Stroke, intracranial hemorrhage, & visual impairment
Young sickle cell patients are at special risk for a life-threatening complication that begins with shock. What is it?	Sequestration crisis *(Presentation is shock & left-sided abdominal mass in a young sickle cell patient)*
What test should initially be ordered for suspected sickle cell disease?	CBC with peripheral blood smear
What follow-up test should be ordered if the initial blood smear suggests sickle cell?	Hemoglobin electrophoresis
What findings on CBC suggest sickle cell?	Anemia Leukocytosis Reticulocytosis >5 %
What findings on peripheral blood smear suggest sickle cell disease?	Sickled cells (surprise!) Howell-Jolly bodies "Helmet" cells
What is a Howell-Jolly body, anyway?	A basophilic inclusion body in the RBC (means the spleen isn't working well, or is missing)
What are the likely causes of bone pain in sickle cell patients?	1. Vasoocclusive infarcts 2. Osteomyelitis 3. AVN

What are the main concerns for sickle cell patients with chest pain?	Pneumonia vs. pulmonary infarcts
Why is hydroxyurea given to sickle cell patients?	To increase the % of fetal hemoglobin (fetal Hgb doesn't sickle)
What blood tests should you generally order for a sickle cell patient presenting in crisis?	CBC Retic count Folate level – optional ESR – optional (CBC & retic count are most essential)
What other diagnostics would you frequently order for sickle cell patients in crisis?	Blood cultures Urine cultures UA X-rays, depending on symptoms
What are the typical therapies used for a patient with SC pain crisis and fever?	1. Hydration 2. Pain mgmt 3. Antibiotic coverage (oxygen was traditionally given, but due to lack of efficacy in some research is no longer standard)
Both xeroderma pigmentosa & albinism are associated with what type(s) of cancer, in general?	Skin cancers (both disorders are autosomal recessive inheritance)
MEN type 1 is associated with development of what type of cancer?	Pancreatic (islet cell) tumors (MEN 1 is pit-para-panc)
MEN type IIa/b is associated with the development of what type(s) of tumors?	1. Medullary ca (both) 2. Pheochromocytoma (both) 3. Mucosal neuromas (IIb) 4. Parathyroid disease (IIa)
Down's syndrome is associated with the development of what type of tumor/cancer?	Leukemia

Tuberous sclerosis causes a variety of problems. What two tumors outside the central nervous system is it related to?	**1. Renal tumors (angiomyolipomas)** **2. Cardiac rhabdomyomas** Mnemonic: Both affected organs have, or start from, "tubes"
Neurofibromatosis, type 1, is associated with two types of oncological diseases. What are they?	**1. Optic pathway glioma** **2. Malignant peripheral nerve sheath tumors**
Neurofibromatosis, type 2, is associated with what bilateral tumor?	**Bilateral acoustic neuromas**
Peutz-Jegher syndrome has perioral freckles and <u>non</u>cancerous GI polyps. What types of cancers are these patients at special risk for? (4)	**1. Gut (stomach & colon)** **2. Breast** **3. Ovarian** **4. Pancreatic**
What is the probability that someone with familial polyposis (of the colon) will develop colon cancer later in life, without treatment?	**100 %**
What unusual type of cancer are retinoblastoma patients at risk for later in life?	**Osteogenic sarcoma**
Turcot syndrome is associated with tumors of a particular organ system. Which organ system gets the tumors?	**CNS**
Turcot syndrome often comes up as a distractor item in test questions. What is Turcot syndrome?	**Familial polyposis** **+** **CNS tumors**
von Hippel-Lindau is associated with several tumors, only one of which is malignant. What malignancy is it?	**Renal cell cancer** (it is also associated with cerebellar hemangiomas & liver/kidney cysts)

Hydrocephalus is rarely due to overproduction of CSF. Which tumor can cause hydrocephalus this way, though?	Choroid plexus papilloma
What is the most common pediatric intracranial tumor?	Cerebellar astrocytoma
Tumor due to amplification of the N-myc oncogene?	Neuroblastoma
Name two types of intracranial tumors that actually occur more often in the PNS?	Neuroblastoma & Schwannoma
Which tumor is most often found in the pineal gland?	Germinoma
Which type of tumor often causes obstructive hydrocephalus at the cerebral aqueduct?	Germinoma
Which type of cerebellar tumor is often associated with retinal and other tumors?	Hemangioblastoma
Which tumor has hallmark "foamy cells" on histology?	Hemangioblastoma
In general, do primary CNS tumors metastasize outside the CNS?	No
Which tumor can metastasize through the CSF? – a very unusual behavior!	Medulloblastoma
15 % of all pediatric CNS tumors are which somewhat scary type of tumor?	Medulloblastoma (it is a common cause of posterior fossa tumors)
Medulloblastoma is highly sensitive to what sort of treatment?	Radiation

What sort of cell does a medulloblastoma come from?	Primitive neural cell precursors
In children, this tumor usually develops in the 4th ventricle, but in adolescents & adults, it is usually found in the spinal cord or cauda equina. Which tumor is it?	Ependymoma
What percentage of brain tumors are glial vs. non-glial?	50 % (but ¾ of *malignant* tumors are glial)
Which CNS tumor is especially associated with von Hippel-Lindau syndrome?	Hemangioblastoma
In kids, 70 % of CNS tumors are _____? (general location)	Infratentorial
In adults, 70 % of tumors are _____? (general location)	Supratentorial
Lymph nodes affected by lymphoma have what characteristics on physical exam?	Firm & rubbery
Lymph node infection presents differently from oncological disease. How?	Nodes are tender and erythematous, and have surrounding edema

Chapter 5
Selected Nephrology Topics

Kidney and Urinary Embryology

It's a good idea to refresh your memory on the basics of kidney development, because it makes remembering and understanding malformations of the kidney much easier. You don't need the details about embryological development, though, for your boards.

There are three phases of embryological kidney development:

1. The **pro**nephros – a very rudimentary kidney develops that is similar to that of primitive fish. It never functions in human embryos.
2. The **meso**nephros – the same type of kidney found in (modern) fish and amphibians. It functions briefly in the human embryo prior to development of the next type of kidney.
3. The **meta**nephros – this kidney starts developing at about 5 weeks of gestational age and begins to make urine at about 12 weeks. It will develop into the adult human kidney.

Origin of the Kidneys

Kidneys develop from two embryological structures.

1. The metanephric diverticulum (aka ureteric bud) – this structure forms the ureter, renal pelvis, calyces, & collecting tubules. It penetrates the adjacent tissue (the metanephric mesoderm), to induce formation of the metanephric cap.
2. The metanephric mesoderm – forms the nephrons.

A uriniferous tubule is defined as a nephron from the metanephric mesoderm and a collecting tubule from the metanephric diverticulum.

© Springer Science+Business Media New York 2016
C.M. Houser, *Pediatric Tricky Topics, Volume 2*,
DOI 10.1007/978-1-4939-3109-5_5

The end of each collecting tubule induces formation of metanephric vesicles, and then tubules of the nephron, in adjacent tissue. The glomeruli invaginate into these tubules.

Kidney Function

During fetal life, the purpose of the kidney is to simply produce urine. Metabolic processing that would normally be done by the kidney is done entirely by the placenta during fetal development.

The production of urine supplies the fetus with much of the amniotic fluid. It is essential that the fetus swallow amniotic fluid to keep the amount of fluid in balance, and to foster proper development of the organs, especially the gastrointestinal system.

Oligohydramnios (very little water) – less amniotic fluid than normal. Results from bilateral renal agenesis or dysfunctional kidney, or from genitourinary obstruction (such as a posterior urethral valve in male infants).

Polyhydramnios (much water) – more amniotic fluid than normal. Results from any type of GI obstruction that prevents the fetus from swallowing amniotic fluid (including anencephaly), or from absorbing it into the fetal gut. Because the fluid is not swallowed and reabsorbed by the GI tract, the total amount of fluid increases. Overproduction of urine can also lead to polyhydramnios. This sometimes occurs with diabetic mothers, due to fetal hyperglycemia & the resulting polyuria. Bartter syndrome, in which urine is overproduced due to altered function in the (renal) loop of Henle.

Kidney Migration & Blood Supply

Kidneys start in the pelvis, very close together, and then move up and out into the abdomen. They also rotate during this process – the hilum starts out pointing directly ventral (down), but rotates clockwise to point medially when they end up in the retroperitoneal space.

At about 9 weeks, the kidneys "run into" the adrenal glands and the glands attach to the top of the kidneys.

The blood supply is initially from the common iliacs. As the kidneys migrate upward into the abdomen, new vessels grow from the aorta and the old vessels disappear. 25 % of adult kidneys have 2–4 renal arteries (extra arteries) that enter the kidney directly – if present these arteries are "end arteries" not collateral circulation. If these arteries are cut or ligated, renal ischemia will result.

Kidney Malformations

Renal agenesis – unilateral occurs 1 per 1,000 live births, bilateral occurs 0.3 per 1,000 live births (more rare, fortunately). Occurs when the metanephric diverticulum doesn't develop, deteriorates, or doesn't invaginate into the metanephric mesoderm. In the end, no nephrons are formed.

Ectopic kidneys – usually in the pelvis – hilar orientation may also be abnormal because the kidney has not rotated during migration.

There is an association between pelvic kidneys and fused kidneys. When the kidneys are in the pelvis they are very close together. If they complete their development there, they sometimes fuse producing one large kidney. (This kidney is usually disc shaped.) Occasionally, a fused kidney migrates to normal position.

Horseshoe kidneys – Horseshoe kidney occurs when one pole of the two kidneys fuses – usually the inferior pole. These kidneys are often found low in the abdomen as they get "caught" under the inferior mesenteric artery (IMA) during the attempted migration process (because they are solid in the middle instead of separated). Horseshoe kidneys are usually asymptomatic but are sometimes prone to obstruction/infection.

Duplication of upper urinary tract – Duplication of the ureters and renal pelvices can occur due to various divisions of the metanephric diverticulum during development. *A truly duplicated whole kidney is rare and probably only occurs if two metanephric diverticula develop.*

Ectopic ureteral orifice – Rare – usually the ureteric orifice is lower than expected and not within the bladder. In females, if the ureter inserts directly into the vagina, parents complain that their daughters' diapers and underwear are continuously wet (incontinence).

Congenital bilateral polycystic kidney – multiple cysts form in the kidney during development which can result in severe renal insufficiency. The cysts are thought to result from abnormal development of the collecting tubules.

LOWER URINARY TRACT DEVELOPMENT

The urorectal septum invaginates into the cloaca forming the rectum and urethra (initially the urogenital sinus).

The urethra has three parts:

1) Vesical – continuous with the allantois. Becomes the urachus, then median umbilical ligament in the adult.
2) Pelvic.
3) Phallic – urogenital membrane covers this portion externally.

The urethral epithelium comes from urogenital sinus endoderm. (The urogenital sinus is the embryological tissue common to both sexes that eventually differentiates into external genitalia and associated structures.) The rest of the urethral tissue comes from "splanchnic mesenchyme," a type of mesoderm adjacent to the epithelium.

The transitional epithelium of the bladder is derived from endoderm from the urogenital sinus – the rest of the bladder develops from the mesoderm.

Note: The bladder is an abdominal organ (whether full or empty) until puberty. After puberty it is ordinarily within the pelvic brim.

Urethral Malformations

Urachal fistula or sinus – This occurs when the urachus remains patent, or when one end or the other is not completely closed forming a blind-ended pouch (sinus). Patients may complain of urine, or simply fluid, leaking from the umbilicus.

Urachal cysts – This occurs when a portion of the midpart of the urachus does not completely close. A small pouch is then formed. Approximately 1/3 of adults have urachal cysts. They are asymptomatic unless they become infected.

Bladder exstrophy – This occurs when the inferior abdominal wall fails to close revealing the anterior portion of the bladder wall and the ureteric orifice area. The anterior bladder wall usually ruptures during birth. Babies are placed on prophylactic antibiotics until surgical repair is performed. It is important to note that bladder exstrophy may be associated with epispadias or lower spinal cord defects.

Epispadias – The urethra does not develop to its full, usual length, and the urethral meatus opens on dorsal or lateral surface of the penis, in its mild form. In the more severe form, it is combined with bladder exstrophy. The basic mechanism for bladder exstrophy & epispadias is thought to be the same (failure of fusion).

Hypospadias – The urethral meatus opens on ventral surface of the penis. The cause is multifactorial involving endocrine, genetic, and environmental factors, and not well understood. The incidence is increased in small-for-gestational-age infants, and infants for whom assisted reproductive technology (especially intracytoplasmic sperm injection – ICSI) was utilized.

Posterior urethral valve (PUV) – In male embryological development, the caudal (tail) end of the Wolffian duct should fuse into the posterior urethral area, forming a collection of folds (plicae colliculi). If the duct does not fuse, but instead forms separate tissue that stretches across the urethral area, a posterior urethral valve is formed. The obstruction it causes in GU outflow both during development often leads to both bladder & kidney abnormalities (as well as secondary effects on lung development).

ADRENAL DEVELOPMENT

Medulla – develops from neural crest cells

Cortex – develops from mesoderm – very large relative to kidney size in fetus and infants – the cortical zones begin to develop late in fetal life and are not completely developed until after birth.

Congenital adrenal hyperplasia – This condition occurs when certain cortical enzymes are deficient, so that some steroid hormones cannot be produced. ACTH is therefore oversecreted (from the pituitary), hyperstimulating the gland and causing hyperplasia.

Hypoplastic adrenals – Occurs in anencephalic infants due to lack of ACTH production and adrenal gland stimulation. The pituitary gland is absent or poorly developed in these infants, so there is no source for ACTH production.

Multicystic vs. Polycystic Kidney Disease

Most physicians are much more familiar with polycystic kidney disease than we are with multicystic kidneys. Multicystic kidneys are an especially important topic, though, for neonatology & pediatric nephrology. This document provides a quick summary comparison of the two disorders.

Polycystic kidney disease

Polycystic kidney disease is an inherited disorder. There are two modes of inheritance, autosomal dominant and autosomal recessive.

Both kidneys are affected in either type of polycystic kidney disease.

The natural history of polycystic kidney disease is that the kidney architecture and function begin relatively normal. As time goes by, the number of cysts increases until kidney function is compromised. In the recessive disorder, this occurs early in childhood, but in the dominant disorder it doesn't occur until well into adulthood.

Multicystic kidney disease

Multicystic kidney disease is a congenital disorder (present at birth) but it is *not* inherited. It results from mechanical problems in the urological system that occur during embryological/fetal development. Most commonly, there is no ureter on the affected side. Multicystic kidneys often have dysplastic tissue (tissue that wouldn't normally occur in the kidney), and always have abnormal architecture. Kidneys that have both cysts and dysplastic tissue are designated to have "multicystic dysplastic kidney disease."

Multicystic kidney disease is usually *unilateral*.

Multicystic kidney disease is the most common cause of an abdominal mass in a newborn, overall (both genders combined).

The natural history of multicystic kidney disease is that the affected kidney is non-functional from birth. No normal parenchymal tissue can be identified in multicystic kidneys – the entire kidney is replaced by non-communicating large cysts.

The contralateral kidney should be evaluated for normal urological function in children with a multicystic kidney. This is because up to 30 % will have reflux on the unaffected side. Untreated reflux could compromise kidney function in the sole functioning kidney if reflux-related complications develop over time.

The treatment of multicystic kidneys is a matter of some controversy. Children with multicystic kidneys are at increased risk for development of renin-mediated hypertension, as well as renal malignancies arising from the scattered stromal cells in the cystic kidney. Some physicians surgically remove the multicystic kidney (nephrectomy), but most currently advocate close monitoring with yearly renal ultrasounds, because the dysplastic kidney typically regresses fully by adolescence.

Amyloidosis: The Essentials

While amyloid disorders do not occur often in pediatrics, they do occur. They are most commonly seen in dialysis patients (usually after about 10 years of dialysis), patients with chronic inflammatory conditions including both rheumatologic disorders & chronic infectious diseases, and rarely in association with certain malignancies. They are uncommon enough to be interesting targets for board examinations & ward discussion of "zebra" disorders.

It is important to understand that amyloid is an amorphous, eosinophilic, protein-aceous substance that can develop from a variety of other molecules in the body. These include immunoglobulin, calcitonin, serum protein, and insulin or glucagon. This material is deposited in a variety of tissues, usually extracellularly, and can cause a number of different problems. **Amyloidosis** refers to the whole group of disorders caused by deposits of proteinaceous, eosinophilic, extracellular material. The tissue the amyloid is ultimately deposited in depends on its molecule of origin.

Amyloidosis that is not linked to another disease or inflammatory state is termed **"primary amyloidosis."** Most of these disorders are late onset & seen in the adult population. Primary amyloidosis mainly affects the heart, tongue, and muscle.

"Secondary amyloidosis" refers to the same problem when it results from a certain serum protein that is present in patients with autoimmune and chronic inflammatory conditions (such as rheumatoid conditions and long-term infections like TB & leprosy). This form is mainly deposited in tissues of the reticuloendothelial system – liver, spleen, lymph nodes, & kidney. Amyloid deposition is also seen in islet cells with type II DM, long-term renal dialysis, and cancers such as medullary thyroid carcinomas.

A newer classification based on the specific molecule in a particular patient's amyloid is now in use. For dialysis patients, this type is β2M-globulin amyloidosis. For most other pediatric patients, the type is "AA." In nations with well-resourced healthcare systems, the frequency of AA due to chronic infectious diseases, as well as disorders such as juvenile idiopathic arthritis (formerly juvenile rheumatoid arthritis), has decreased due to better recognition & management of those disorders. The most common etiologies for AA amyloidosis in the pediatric populations of those countries now are thought to be autoimmune disorders, and in particular, familial Mediterranean fever.

While less of an issue during the pediatric period, Down's syndrome patients invariably develop amyloid deposition in later life in the central nervous system, producing an early-onset type of Alzheimer's dementia.

The structure of amyloid is always a β-pleated sheet. Buzzwords in the diagnosis of amyloidosis are **Congo red dye** (a dye that it absorbs) and **apple green birefringence** (its appearance under polarized light microscopy).

Word associations that you may find useful:

AMYLOID --- β-PLEATED SHEETS --- CONGO RED DYE --- APPLE GREEN BIREFRINGENCE

AMYLOID --- PRIMARY --- IG --- HEART, MUSCLE, TONGUE --- PLASMA CELL DISEASES

AMYLOID --- SECONDARY --- AA TYPE --- CHRONIC INFLAMMATION --- SERUM PROTEIN --- LIVER, KIDNEY, SPLEEN

AMYLOID – SECONDARY – RENAL DIALYSIS – LONG TERM -- β2M-GLOBULIN TYPE

AMYLOID β-PROTEIN – ALZHEIMER'S DISEASE --- CHROMOSOME 21

Fluids and Electrolytes: Critical Care and Boards Topics

Sodium

Sodium is the main thing (or at least the main electrolyte) that determines extracellular fluid volume (ECFV). It is also the main extracellular cation (potassium is the main *intra*cellular cation).

Regulating sodium is an important way to regulate ECFV – what we normally think of as the patient's "volume status."

Total body sodium – How is it regulated?

1. **Kidney juxtaglomerular cells** notice if renal perfusion decreases – they release renin $\rightarrow$ angiotensin $\rightarrow$ angiotensin I $\rightarrow$ angiotensin II

   Angiotensin II tells the kidney to retain more sodium than usual, *and* causes release of aldosterone --

   Released by the adrenal cortex, aldosterone also increases the amount of sodium the kidney retains (rather than excreting the sodium into the urine, Na is absorbed in the collecting duct).

2. **Volume sensors in the atria and great veins** notice if volume is unusually high – if it is, they cause release of atrial natriuretic factor (ANF) from the heart. ANF increases sodium excretion (dumps sodium out of the body – like aldosterone, ANF also acts on the collecting duct, but this time it prevents absorption of sodium).

   (This makes sense because "atrial" refers to the atrium, which is monitoring the volume status, while "natri" refers to sodium, and "uretic" refers to urinary excretion, like in the word "diuretic.")

3. **Low-volume sensors in the carotid sinus and aorta** activate the sympathetic nervous system – producing more renin release, and sodium retention by the kidney.

Total body water – How is it regulated (by the kidney, that is)?

1. Adequate GFR (glomerular filtration rate) must be available
2. Adequate delivery of fluid to the glomerulous must happen
3. Kidney must be working properly (able to concentrate or dilute – a healthy kidney is able to concentrate or dilute urine until the GFR reaches 20 % of normal)
4. ADH system must work (turns on and off correctly)
5. Kidney is responding properly to ADH

In addition to the total body water, other contributors to ECFV are as follows:

Thirst/tonicity – Hypertonicity is the main trigger for thirst and ADH release. (Hypertonicity is defined as the ability of the solutes in a solution to generate an osmotic driving force for water movement.)

ADH status:

The most important factor in determining whether concentrated or dilute urine is produced is ADH (antidiuretic hormone – made by the pituitary).

Lack of ADH (centrally) is *central* diabetes insipidus (DI).

Kidney unresponsiveness to ADH is *nephrogenic* DI.

Drugs or conditions with ADH-like effects, or that increase ADH→SIADH syndrome.

Potassium

Remember that potassium is the main intracellular cation (only 3.5–5.0 mEq/L *outside* cells, but 130–140 mEq/L *inside* cells).

How are appropriate potassium levels maintained?

Basic mechanisms:

Regular body cells maintain their potassium gradient with a Na-K ATPase pump.

Dietary potassium is handled by the kidney and the gut –
Kidney – 90 % of dietary K is excreted in urine
Gut – 10 % of dietary K is excreted in stool

The kidney can dump up to 10 mEq/kg/24 h, if necessary. Needless to say, *hyperkalemia rarely develops when kidney function is normal*. The kidney maintains its ability to dump potassium until it is down to only 20 % of its regular function!

Kidney cells (of the collecting duct) are set up to allow secretion of one K ion into the urine, with resorption of one Na ion. This means that the more K is dumped in the urine, the greater the sodium retention will be.

Clinically, if less sodium is sitting in the collecting duct, as often happens in the newborn period due to low sodium content in formula or breast milk, then less K will be secreted, increasing serum K levels.

Other modifying factors:

Gut – much more potassium (than the usual 10 % of dietary potassium) can be dumped via the gut *if* the serum is hyperkalemic, and also with diarrhea
Insulin – drives K *inside* cells
Acidosis – drives K *out of* cells, *and* decreases renal excretion of K (generally) (because the collecting duct secretes H ions instead of K ions in an effort to decrease the acidosis)
Alkalosis – drives K *inside* cells, *and* increases renal excretion of K (generally)
β-2 receptor stimulation – drives K *inside* cells (remember that albuterol can be used to temporarily decrease the plasma K level, because it is a beta-2 agonist)
Increased serum osmolality – brings K *out of* cells (remember that increased osmolality means increased solutes compared to the fluid volume – the solutes that determine osmolality are sodium (main determinant), glucose, and urea)

Why?
1. As cells dehydrate, the K concentration inside the cell gets higher, pushing some of the K to leave the cell.
2. Solvent drag – As water exits the cell due to the high osmolality outside it, some of the solutes are literally just drug out of the cell with the water.

Aldosterone – lowers potassium because it increases potassium loss in the urine (aldosterone release is stimulated by hyperkalemia, as well as the renin-angiotensin system)

How? It upregulates the number of Na/K exchangers in the collecting tubule. It also increases Na channel activity. Together, this increases Na absorption from the tubular lumen – K secretion goes up so that one positive ion goes out for each positive ion taken in (electroneutrality).

High sodium load – The more sodium is presented to the collecting tubule, the more potassium is excreted (because more sodium/potassium exchange is possible, and encouraged, by the presence of so much sodium!).

Poorly resorbed anions – These anions, including excess bicarb, carry sodium and water (the water comes along due to osmosis) into the collecting tubule. For example, sodium can be transported across as sodium bicarb. Higher flow in the collecting duct due to the increased water volume further stimulates K secretion through a mechanism known as "flow-dependent K secretion."

Sweating – It is possible to lose a significant amount of potassium through sweating, but only if the volume of sweat is really large!

DKA Question that illustrates some of these mechanisms:

If acidosis *decreases* renal excretion of potassium, why do DKA patients often become dangerously hypokalemic?

Answer: First, the hypovolemia that develops in DKA leads to aldosterone secretion. Aldosterone upregulates the Na/K channels of the collecting tubule, leading to increased potassium loss, in an effort to preserve sodium, the main determinant of adequate blood volume.

Second, the volume loss of DKA is mainly due to the osmotic diuresis induced by so much circulating glucose. The excess glucose delivered to the kidney brings a lot more water than usual with it. As the glucose crosses into the kidney tubules, the water osmotically follows. This produces an unusually high flow rate in the tubule, stimulating "flow-dependent K secretion" by the collecting duct, and increasing urinary loss of potassium.

Bicarbonate

Remember that the ABG bicarb value is *calculated – not measured!*

The kidney resorbs almost all filtered bicarb in the proximal tubule, *if* bicarb is in the normal range. This does not affect the pH at all – bicarb has not been added, merely reclaimed.

If you think about it, resorption of the usual circulating bicarb needs to be very close to complete – otherwise metabolic acidosis would slowly develop, due to decreasing circulating bicarb.

If there is an unusually large amount of circulating bicarb, though, as in metabolic alkalosis, the excess bicarb will spill into the urine (helping to correct the alkalosis).

How the kidney finds bicarb for the body, if extra bicarb is needed (for example, with long-term acidosis):

1. The main mechanism is hydrolysis of the amino acid glutamine. This produces two NH4+ (also known as ammonium), and two bicarb molecules that will be absorbed into the bloodstream.
2. Active H+ secretion – one bicarb can be retrieved for each H+ secreted (this is a normal, baseline process – it allows the body to recover bicarb, but bicarb is not generated as part of this process).

(Note: Defective H+ elimination is the reason for type I (distal) RTA – In this disorder, HCO3- is used up binding the excess acid, producing acidosis.)

How is bicarb resorption determined?

1. Low circulating volume – *increases* bicarb resorption (proximal tubule does it)
2. Increased angiotensin II – *increases* bicarb resorption (proximal tubule)
3. Increased PCO2 – *increases* bicarb resorption, while low PCO2 decreases it
4. Low total body potassium – *increases* bicarb resorption, while high total body potassium decreases bicarb resorption

(Note: Defective proximal tubule resorption of bicarb is type II (proximal) RTA.)

The mysterious "contraction alkalosis":

There is nothing mysterious about contraction alkalosis (contraction refers to a low circulating volume). Low volume means increased proximal tubule resorption of HCO3-, encouraging a metabolic alkalosis – but the actual effect on the patient's pH is small.

To explain this in more detail … when you have a low circulatory volume, aldosterone and angiotensin II increase. Aldosterone causes some potassium wasting, through its action on the "principal" cells in the kidney. In compensation, it also stimulates H/K exchangers in the collecting duct, which helps to recover some of the body's K. (Severe hypokalemia affects the resting membrane potential in skeletal muscle, cardiac muscle, brain cells, etc. It hyperpolarizes them, making it difficult for them to reach their threshold for activity.) When K ions are reabsorbed into the collecting duct cells, H ions are exchanged for them. The H/K ion exchange preserves electroneutrality for the body, but the excess free H ions are lost in the urine, contributing to alkalosis. In addition, angiotensin II stimulates increased bicarbonate reabsorption by the proximal tubular cells directly, augmenting the alkalosis.

Other alkalosis:

Don't forget that nasogastric suctioning is just like vomiting – it can also cause a metabolic alkalosis.

Certain diuretics, such as thiazides and loop diuretics, also tend to cause metabolic alkalosis through a "contracted" volume state (activating aldosterone and angiotensin II). These medications also tend to cause potassium loss through "flow-dependent K secretion" in the collecting duct.

Does volume expansion cause "expansion acidosis?"

Theoretically, yes. Once again, the effect is usually small, and most patients who require volume expansion are much more in need of a blood pressure than the perfect pH. Basically, the idea is that rapid volume expansion with fluids that lack bicarb could dilute the bicarb initially present in the patient's bloodstream, causing a temporary acidosis. Additionally, volume expansion turns off secretion of aldosterone and angiotensin II.

Anion-Gap Acidosis

If H+ is joined to an anion that is not measured by our usual lab tests, and that molecule is present in the body, it increases the anion gap. The normal anion gap (sodium – (bicarb + chloride)) is about 10–14.

All acidoses that are not purely respiratory are, by exclusion, at least partly a metabolic acidosis. Even if you add a toxin, as in a toxic ingestion, it is still considered a "metabolic acidosis."

The higher the anion gap, the more likely it is that there is an underlying metabolic acidosis, even if it is being compensated for by the kidney or respiratory system.

Normal-anion Gap Acidosis (also known as Non-anion Gap Acidosis)

If your patient is acidotic, and their anion gap is normal, you will sometimes hear that the patient has a "hyperchloremic" acidosis. Why?

Because an acidotic patient will usually have a lower than normal bicarb. (Remember that the patient's bicarb should be busy taking up hydrogen ions.). If the anion gap is normal in an acidotic patient, it is usually because the chloride ion is high, which makes up for the lack of bicarb when you do the calculation.

Clinically, the most common reasons for a patient's normal anion gap metabolic acidosis are RTA or diarrhea.

Hypernatremia – How Does It Happen?

The cause is usually water deficit.
Water deficit can develop from:
- Loss of H_2O from the kidney, or from non-kidney sources such as fever/heat, hyperventilation, or diarrhea
- Failure to replace H_2O (marathon runners who don't drink enough replacement fluids)
- Iatrogenic addition of sodium (rare)

When hypernatremia develops from non-renal causes, the patients often have a decreased total body sodium, in addition to a decreased volume status overall.

Why is hypernatremia a problem? Mainly because the shrinking (dehydrated) brain puts tension on the bridging vessels, and sometimes causes intracranial bleeding if those vessels tear.

Alert people who can feel thirst and get water don't become hypernatremic! (This is why the elderly are more at risk, their thirst mechanism is decreased, and sometimes it is difficult for them to get their own fluids. Children, of course, are often in the same position.) If your patient is hypernatremic, there is an underlying cause – change of mental status, neurological disease, unable to independently conduct activities of daily living, etc.

When might the kidney cause hypernatremia?
Basically, when there is a *high osmotic load*, or when *central or nephrogenic diabetes insipidus* is the trouble. In pediatrics, nephrocalcinosis is an important cause, especially in low-birth-weight neonates. Hypernatremia develops because the (medullary) kidney isn't able to concentrate the urine very well, leading to unusually high body water loss.

Causes of osmotic diuresis – diabetes (glucose), hyperalimentation (due to high urea load from catabolism of high-protein diets), mannitol (usually given as a temporary way to try to decrease ICP or intraocular pressure)

How will you know whether the cause of polyuria is osmotic diuresis or DI?
Aside from history information, you can look at the osmolality of the urine. This sounds like something difficult to remember, but it's really not.
Very high osmolality goes with osmotic diuresis. (This makes sense – high osmolality means that there's a lot of stuff in the urine. Osmotic diuresis happens because there's a lot of stuff in the bloodstream that is ending up in the urine.)

Typical osmolality for an osmotic diuresis will be above 300 mOsm/L.
Typical osmolality for a DI diuresis is low – less than 150 mOsm/L.

Remember that diabetes insipidus occurs when either the central nervous system fails to produce ADH (aka vasopressin) or the kidney fails to respond to the ADH it encounters. The CNS failing to make ADH is "central" diabetes insipidus. The kidney failing to respond to ADH is "nephrogenic" diabetes insipidus. (Makes sense again!)

If the kidney can't reabsorb free water to concentrate the urine, of course the osmolality will be low!

There is one other unusual way DI can develop – psychogenic polydipsia. Psychogenic polydipsia is when a patient drinks too much free water due to a psychiatric disorder. In its extreme form, the amount of free water the kidney tries to filter for the patient *actually washes out the medullary gradient over time!* The patient is left with an unusual form of DI, until the patient's free water can be restricted, and the gradient recreated by the kidney.

How is hypernatremia treated?
Slowly – rapid correction causes the brain to swell!

Correct volume first – use NS until the patient maintains a good blood pressure. You can then use hypotonic solutions, but be careful that you don't lower the sodium more than

$$0.5 \text{ mEq/L/h or no more than } 10 \text{ mEq/L per day}$$

While it is clinically not really important, as you will be frequently checking labs, it is good to know the formula for water deficit if you will be going on ICU rounds. It is not tough.

H20 deficit = Total body water × (amount of sodium is off/normal sodium)
(total body water is conservatively calculated as about .5 × total body weight)

By the way, use the patient's normal body weight, as you are trying to get them back to that weight, not the shriveled-like-a-raisin weight they currently have.

Hyponatremia

The usual cause of hyponatremia is continued free water intake, while renal excretion of water is impaired.

Remember that as with all changes in sodium concentration, it is the *rate of change* that determines the symptoms, not the sodium level itself.

Texts usually describe three types of hyponatremia. All of them have long, scary sounding names. Fortunately, the ideas behind the names are straightforward.

Hyponatremia is categorized based on the tonicity of the patient's serum. How do we measure tonicity? Serum osmolality.

Hyponatremia with Hypertonicity

This problem occurs in specific situations, such as administration of mannitol, or very high glucose, as in DKA. The total body sodium amount is fine, but the concentration in the serum is low, because the serum is full of some other solute. The other solute causes the hypertonicity.

The most common cause of hyponatremia with hypertonicity is high glucose in diabetics. Remember that the correction to determine the actual sodium level without all that solute is to increase the sodium value by 1.6 for every 100 mg/dL glucose exceeds its normal value of 100.

Hypertonic hyponatremia does not cause symptoms of hyponatremia, because the total circulating sodium is actually fine (normal).

This type of hyponatremia is often appropriately called "pseudohyponatremia," although historically pseudohyponatremia should refer to the normal tonicity condition described next.

Pseudohyponatremia (Hyponatremia with Normal Tonicity)
With modern laboratory techniques, this situation is rarely seen in current clinical practice. Pseudohyponatremia occurs when either triglycerides or proteins are very high in the serum (for example, in some cases of multiple myeloma). This falsely lowers the sodium concentration obtained on lab tests, depending on the technology used in the lab. In other words, this is basically the same situation as hyponatremia with hypertonicity, except that proteins and triglycerides do not significantly alter the tonicity of the serum.

Hyponatremia with Hypotonicity (True Hyponatremia)
This is the most common type of hyponatremia. It results from impaired renal water excretion, with continued normal water intake.

How does true hyponatremia happen?

1. Kidney failure to less than 20 % GFR.
2. Hypovolemia – The kidney won't excrete water, despite low sodium, because the overall volume is low. This is seen with persistent vomiting, marathon runners who won't replenish fluids, etc.
3. SIADH (associated with neuro and pulmonary conditions, remember).
4. Adrenal insufficiency – poor sodium retention without aldosterone.
5. Thiazide diuretics – they specifically block the kidney's ability to excrete free water, even though their overall effect is diuresis.
6. Hypothyroidism – reasons are "complex," but it sometimes happens.
7. Very limited diet (severe solute restriction) – due to a decreased ability to excrete excess H2O. Also seen with very serious beer drinking (the only solute is carbohydrate, and it turns into water and CO2!).
8. Edematous states (sometimes) – despite increased salt retention, some edema patients eventually become hyponatremic, given the excess water their body is storing.

How is True Hyponatremia Treated (Generally)?
The mainstay of treatment is water restriction. The other mainstay of treatment is that correction should be slow. Why? Because the brain stem is a terrible thing to waste! *Central pontine myelinolysis*, also known as *"osmostic demyelination syndrome,"* can cause permanent neurological sequelae.

What do I need to know about central pontine myelinolysis?
It develops from overly rapid correction of hyponatremia.

It usually develops a day or more *after* the sodium has been corrected.

The typical symptoms are change of mental status, problems with swallowing, loss of vision, quadriplegia, and seizures. (For patients in extremis & with ongoing seizures, 3 % saline can be given to raise the sodium just high enough to end the seizures. This is an area in which the recommendations change regularly, however.)

Patients at greatest risk of CPM are the chronically ill, including cancer patients, and those who have recently had a cardiac arrest.

How is True Hyponatremia Treated (Specifically)?

Edematous hyponatremia – If your edematous patient is also hyponatremic, then both water *and sodium* should be restricted. (In your usual edema patient, you restrict sodium only.) Certain diuretics will also help with the total body sodium overload.

Clinically, edematous hyponatremia is seen in patients with minimal change disease (MCD). Fluid and salt restriction is the appropriate initial MCD treatment while waiting for response to the main treatment, which is steroids. (Diuretics for edema, & NSAIDs to decrease proteinuria, are sometimes also given.)

Question: Which class of diuretics must you avoid in hyponatremia?

Thiazides – they block formation of dilute urine. Thiazides will reduce the edema, but they will also worsen the hyponatremia.

Hypokalemia

Remember that, as with many other conditions, hypokalemia can be "real" or it can be a consequence of potassium shifting out of the bloodstream. In this case, the total body potassium is fine, but the measured value is low.

A few unusual causes of hypokalemia that you should be aware of are:
Familial hypokalemic periodic paralysis (aka periodic paralysis)
     This is an autosomal dominant disorder in which the potassium sometimes drops precipitously – often at night. The mechanism is not clear, and no life-threatening problems of hypokalemia develop.

Megaloblastic anemia – when treatment begins
When treatment begins for megaloblastic anemia (vitamin supplementation) RBCs are produced very quickly. A significant amount of potassium is needed to "stock" the intracellular potassium supply for the red blood cells. The sudden use of potassium for the new RBCs will sometimes drop the serum potassium enough to require supplementation.

Bartter's syndrome
This is a very rare disorder in which renin and aldosterone are increased, with low potassium and metabolic alkalosis. The syndrome most often results from a

mutation that causes "chronic Lasix-like picture." Patients with Bartter's syndrome can't generate the renal medullary gradient needed to produce concentrated urine. The high urinary flow rate of Bartter's syndrome leads to hypokalemia via the "flow-dependent K secretion" mechanism. It is treated with potassium, potassium-sparing diuretics, and NSAIDs, because they tend to decrease potassium loss in the urine.

(The inability to concentrate urine also leads to volume depletion, of course, and contraction alkalosis.)

Can poor potassium intake cause hypokalemia?
Essentially, no. The kidneys are very good at preserving potassium.

What does a hypokalemic patient look like?
Hypokalemic patients have weak muscles, and sometimes develop rhabdomyolysis.

The muscles of the gut don't work well without potassium either – patients develop ileus and constipation.

Polyuria occurs in some patients, when potassium is low. (This occurs due to increased dilation of the afferent arteriole of the glomerulus in low-potassium states. More dilation means more fluid in the glomerulus being filtered, & higher quantities of urine production.)

The most dreaded complication, of course, is arrhythmia. Remember that hypokalemic arrhythmia often *does not* respond to defibrillation. Remember also that digoxin + hypokalemia increases the patients' chances of having a serious arrhythmia!

So, once again, that's weak skeletal muscles, weak GI muscles, weak/unpredictable heart muscle, and sometimes polyuria.

If intake isn't the problem, why do patients become hypokalemic?
There are a bunch of reasons – here we go …

Diarrhea – Bicarb is lost in diarrhea, *but so is potassium.*

Magnesium depletion – Somehow, if magnesium is low, it prevents either potassium or calcium from achieving normal values

Alkalosis – makes potassium hide in the cells – total body potassium is not affected.

β-2 agonists – increase the activity of Na-K ATPase channels on the cell membranes. This tends to decrease the circulating potassium – total body potassium is not affected.

Certain medications – Some medications encourage hypokalemia, mainly by increasing flow rate in the collecting duct. As discussed above, this stimulates K secretion into the urine via "flow-dependent K secretion."

Metabolic acidosis (certain types) – Certain types of metabolic acidosis cause loss of potassium. This might be confusing, at first, as alkalosis lowers the serum level of potassium. The changes we see in potassium level with acidosis, though, reflect the real loss of potassium ions – not just a shift of potassium into cells. Through various mechanisms, the metabolic acidosis conditions that lose potassium are:
DKA (osmotic diuresis loss)

Ureterosigmoidostomy (K loss due to metabolic derangement in about 80 % of patients)

RTA types I & II (renal changes produce K loss)

Specifically, in a proximal RTA, less bicarb is resorbed. This means that increased amounts of sodium-bicarb form, as the bicarb binds to the sodium already available in the fluid. Sodium bicarb then acts as an osmotic diuretic, and K is lost by, you guessed it, "flow-dependent K secretion."

In a distal RTA, the collecting duct cells don't secrete many H ions, so K ions are secreted instead, leading to hypokalemia.

So, if the patient's hypokalemic, can I just give potassium to fix it?

Yes. Treatment for hypokalemia is usually quite simple. For patients whose EKGs are essentially normal, and who are not in any other extremis, potassium should be supplemented orally. Of course, the reason for the hypokalemia should also be investigated. Any underlying causes need to be identified and corrected.

If the patient requires rapid correction of potassium, it can be given IV – usually in 10–20 mEq slow drips – until a reasonable level is achieved. If the potassium is given too fast, *it can cause fatal arrhythmias*. Additionally, it is very irritating to the veins, and uncomfortable for the patient. (So … patience is a virtue when it comes to K+ delivery.)

Hyperkalemia

When is it really bad? >6.5 mEq/L

What are the usual symptoms & signs?

Muscle weakness, arrhythmias, EKG changes (peaked Ts – like a peak of potassium, flat Ps, prolonged PR interval, wide QRS – heading for a sine wave eventually, if the potassium gets really high)

As with other electrolyte disorders, the first thing to think about with hyperkalemia is whether the high potassium is a real finding, or whether you are being fooled into thinking it is high. This can occur with *pseudo*hyperkalemia (not real hyperkalemia, at all), or when the problem is in the distribution of total body potassium, rather than total body oversupply of potassium (redistribution).

Common causes of *pseudo*hyperkalemia (not real hyperkalemia, at all) are:
Hemolysis during the blood draw (intracellular K is spilled)
Too many platelets or leukocytes will sometimes falsely elevate the K level

Common causes of *redistribution* hyperkalemia are:
Metabolic or respiratory acidosis (H and K are exchanged in an effort to maintain the pH near normal)
Burn injuries, crush injuries, lightning injuries – anything that causes cells to break open.

Hypertonicity – K is sucked out into the bloodstream due to the unusual tonicity

Digitalis overdose – the Na/K ATPase pump is incapacitated by dig. If it is not working, then the usually low potassium levels will rise

Beta-blockers – cause a mild elevation (just as beta-agonists cause a mild depression)

Succinylcholine use – causes potassium levels to increase by about 0.5 mEq due to increased muscle membrane permeability

Familial hyperkalemic periodic paralysis – yes, there is a familial disorder causing periodic paralysis with both transiently high *and* low potassium levels

True hyperkalemia usually develops through one of the four mechanisms:

1. Renal failure (GFR <20 %)
2. Aldosterone deficiency, or an aldosterone-unresponsive kidney (aka RTA type 4)
3. Medications – medications that decrease aldosterone, or interfere with its effects, often cause hyperkalemia (example: NSAIDs, ACE inhibitors, heparin, and potassium-sparing diuretics)
4. Hyporeninemic hypoaldosteronism – a chronic, abnormally low, level of renin secretion produces a chronic hyperkalemia. This problem is most often seen in diabetics

Treatment for hyperkalemia requiring acute intervention:
(In other words, people with EKG changes or arrhythmias)

There are several ways to rapidly decrease potassium levels. Check the EKG to know whether rapid decrease is needed – arrhythmias or EKG changes of hyperkalemia mean *treat now!* If the patient's rhythm deteriorates into one that does not perfuse, it is incredibly difficult to correct in cases of potassium imbalance. You want to treat before the situation becomes that bad.

Treatment options:

1. Beta-agonists – as a stop-gap, they will lower the potassium a bit, for a little while. They are especially important if IV access is not yet established. Inhaled albuterol is usually used.
2. IV push medications – things that chase potassium into the cell are used: insulin (glucose is also given to avoid causing hypoglycemia), and bicarb. Calcium is usually given first to "stabilize" the cardiac membrane, in an effort to reduce the probability of arrhythmia.
3. Dialysis – used if the kidney is not functioning, and if dialysis can be accomplished rapidly (for example, renal failure patients with existing shunts).

Note: Giving kayexalate – Potassium-binding resins such as kayexalate are often given in the acute setting. While there is no harm in giving kayexalate, it will not lower the potassium level very quickly.

Sequence of medication administration in symptomatic patients:

1. For patients with QRS widening or hypotension, calcium is given first, because it is thought to decrease the likelihood of arrhythmias.
2. Give beta-agonists (usually nebulized albuterol) if no IV/IO access is available.
3. IV push glucose with insulin to facilitate K going into the cells (the K is only dangerous when it is extracellular, and circulating in the blood).
4. Give bicarb IV push (shifts pH to facilitate K going intracellular & staying there).

Special cases:

Aldosterone-deficient patients: These patients require a diet low in potassium, as their kidney will not be excreting potassium the way most others do. Loop diuretics are helpful, mainly because high flow to the collecting duct stimulates K secretion.

Fludrocortisone is sometimes used in these patients to replace the missing mineralocorticoids. It is a tricky way to treat, though, as the increased sodium retention it promotes sometimes leads to hypervolemia.

Aldosterone-unresponsive patients: Low potassium diet and loop diuretics. Fludrocortisone won't work in these patients, as the kidney is unresponsive.

Chronic renal failure: Low-potassium diet, loop diuretics if the patient is not anuric, kayexalate (long term), eliminating any hidden sources of potassium in the diet or medications is important, and finally, of course, they can be dialyzed.

Metabolic acidosis

How does metabolic acidosis occur?

1. Increased endogenous acids (e.g., renal failure)
2. Increased exogenous acids (e.g., ingested toxins that produce acids)
3. Decreased excretion of H+ ions (RTA types 1 or IV)
4. Unusually large bicarb losses in the kidney (RTA type II)
5. Unusually large bicarb losses in the gut, typically due to diarrhea

Why do we care about acidosis?

Below a pH of 7.2, the heart begins to lose contractility. Death is a bad outcome. Also, the disorders that cause acidosis are often life threatening.

Acidoses are divided into anion gap and normal-anion gap acidoses. What does it mean?

Anion-gap acidoses occur in two general circumstances. Either a toxin is taken into the body that affects the acid-base balance of the body or an acid produced by the body itself does the same thing. Because the formula requires that we subtract the negative ions chloride and bicarb from the positive ion sodium, the "anion gap" widens to larger than normal as bicarb is used up by the new acid.

The anion gap is important mainly because, when it is present, it gives us a clue to the cause of our patient's pH problem.

What is an example of a normal-anion-gap acidosis?

Mild and moderate levels of renal insufficiency usually produce a normal-anion-gap acidosis. The acidosis occurs because the kidney is not able to produce ammonia as well as it normally would. Ammonia is the main mechanism for renal excretion of hydrogen ions. A second mechanism is the low flow of urine in renal insufficiency, which prevents the usual amount of H ion secretion in the collecting duct.

In an increased anion-gap acidosis, why is the increase in acid not matched 1:1 by a decrease in the bicarb? It should be!

This "discrepancy" occurs because hydrogen ions are buffered by other parts of the body, in addition to the bicarb ions. Bicarb does not need to decrease quite as much as the acid has increased, because H+ is also buffered by bone and inside cells. Bicarb decreases a little less than expected, due to a little help from its friends!

How do you know what the bicarb *should be* in an anion-gap acidosis?

It can be calculated – and it's not even tough to do.

$$\text{Change in AG} = \text{Change in bicarb} \times 1.5.$$

If the change in the bicarb is different from what you would expect, there is probably something else going on.

Higher bicarb than expected indicates that there may be a "hidden" metabolic alkalosis.

Lower bicarb than expected indicates that there may be a "hidden" acidosis (either kind).

Anion-Gap Acidosis Mnemonic (there are many out there, this is just one of them)

Methanol, Metformin	Paraldehyde & paint huffing
Uremia	INH & iron
DKA	Lactic acidosis
	Ethylene glycol & ethanol
	Salicylates & sepsis

Normal-anion-Gap Acidosis Mnemonic (NAGs are HARD UP)

Hypervolemia	Ureterosigmoidostomy
ACE inhibitor	Pancreaticoduodenal fistula
RTA types 1, 2, &4	
Diarrhea	

Specific Types of High Anion-Gap Acidosis

Diabetic ketoacidosis – The quantity of ketones present is often underestimated by the ketone dipstick test. This is because the dipstick only detects the presence of acetoacetate. Another common ketone form, betahydroxybutyrate, is *not measured.* Bear this in mind when checking the ketones of DKA patients. The problem is even worse in alcoholic ketoacidosis.

Alcoholic ketoacidosis – Results from a combination of starving and ethanol-induced changes in the availability of glycogen for energy. Happens faster in small children! As mentioned above, dipstick tests for ketones are notoriously inaccurate in these patients, as *most* of their ketones are in the betahydroxybutyrate form.

Interestingly, alcoholic ketoacidosis patients often have a respiratory alkalosis. Why? They breathe rapidly.

Of further interest, alcoholic ketoacidosis patients often have a mixed acid-base problem because, in addition to ketoacidosis and respiratory alkalosis, they often also have a metabolic alkalosis. Why? They vomit a lot.

Don't let this overwhelm you, just think about the possibilities mentioned above if an alcoholic patient presents with a confusing acid-base set of issues.

Uremic acidosis – High anion-gap acidosis only develops in renal failure when the GFR falls below 20 %. Until then, there is usually a mild non-anion-gap acidosis. Why does the anion gap go up when the kidney is really having trouble? Unmeasured anions such as sulfate, phosphate, and other organic anions are no longer excreted.

Salicylates – Salicylate overdose has an unusual acid-base presentation that is interesting – and *frequently tested*. Early in the overdose, the patient will have a respiratory alkalosis, because salicylates stimulate the CNS breathing center for more rapid breathing. As the metabolic acidosis builds, the pH crosses normal and heads for acidosis.

In addition to the acid of the salicylate itself, much of the acid in salicylate overdoses results from the action it has on body metabolic pathways overall. These metabolic effects tend to produce significant amounts of lactic acids and ketones.

Ethylene glycol – Comes from drinking antifreeze or radiator fluid. Usually seen in alcoholics. It creates an anion-gap acidosis, but also kills the kidneys, producing additional acid issues. The buzzword is "calcium oxalate crystals in the urine." Urine may also fluoresce with a Wood's lamp, due to the colorant added to antifreeze.

Specific Types of Non-Anion-Gap Acidosis (aka normal gap)

Mild-to-moderate renal failure – as mentioned above, as long as the kidney is still able to excrete the "unmeasured anions," a mild NAG acidosis results from renal insufficiency.

Diarrhea can cause a NAG acidosis due to loss of bicarb (don't forget K is also lost).

Distal RTA (type 1): Can't excrete H+ ions – associated with hypokalemia & calcium-based renal stones. Causes of RTA 1 include hyperparathyroidism, Sjogren's, & amphotericin B.

Proximal RTA (type 2): Can't resorb bicarb – one version of RTA 2 is Fanconi's syndrome. In this case, the tubule fails to resorb bicarb, amino acids, glucose, phosphorous, & urate.

The kidney has *no problem* acidifying the urine by excreting H+; it just can't resorb bicarb. Causes of RTA 2 include Wilson disease, Alport disease, and multiple myeloma (in adults, acetazolamide, & heavy metal poisonings).

RTA 4: Don't have, or can't respond to, aldosterone – potassium is always high when this cause of acidosis is present. Patients who lack aldosterone will respond to mineralocorticoid therapy (fludrocortisone). Patients whose kidney cannot respond to aldosterone will not respond to mineralocorticoids, either.

Causes of RTA 4 include sickle cell, obstruction of the GU system, analgesic nephropathy and NSAID use, heparin, ACE inhibitors, and K-sparing diuretics.

A Few Notes on Metabolic Alkalosis

Treatment?
Metabolic alkalosis is usually better tolerated than metabolic acidosis is. Most metabolic alkalosis can be treated with normal saline volume expansion. Alkalosis that develops due to mineralocorticoid excess will *not* respond to normal saline (see below).

The typical cause of metabolic alkalosis is vomiting. Some more exotic reasons follow.

Mineralocorticoid excess – produces alkalosis and hypokalemia, of course. How does it produce alkalosis? Mineralocorticoids increase hydrogen ion secretion in the collecting tubule. This produces metabolic alkalosis over time.

Bartter's syndrome – mentioned above as a cause of hypokalemia, Bartter's syndrome also produces alkalosis. In Bartter's syndrome, renin and aldosterone levels are high, while potassium is low. The main problem is a potassium "leak channel" present on certain renal cells (TALH cells). If this channel doesn't function properly, the Na-Cl-2K transporters also can't work properly – producing the same situation you see when a patient is given Lasix. The diuresis produces hypovolemia, stimulating the renin-aldosterone system to try to preserve circulating intravascular volume. The rush of fluid through the collecting duct produces the usual loss of potassium, due to flow-dependent K secretion.

What is a "mixed" acid-base disorder?

This is a situation with two or more *independent* acid-base disorders occurring. Compensation for an initial acid-base disorder *does not* constitute a mixed disorder.

Ways to figure out whether you're seeing a compensated metabolic disorder, or a "mixed" disorder

Most of the time, you will already have figured out what type of metabolic disorder your patient has, just by looking at the pH, and then seeing whether the CO_2 or the bicarb seems to be responsible for it.

If you feel you need to look into the matter further, however, here is a way to do it. Most of the time, this is not needed. It is also not always possible to determine exactly what the combination of acid-base issues might be. Remember to think about the clinical scenario. Often the history and other information in the case tell you what the acid-base disorder is, rather than the calculations.

Metabolic Alkalosis:

In metabolic alkalosis, pCO_2 should go up, to bring the pH nearer to 7.4. If it's down, you obviously have a respiratory metabolic issue. If it's up, how do you know whether it's up as far as it ought to be?

Step 1: Look at the bicarb, and determine how abnormal it is. For example, if it is 15, it is about 9 point lower than it ought to be.

Step 2: Multiply by 0.7. In this case, 9×0.7 will give you the amount of CO_2 elevation you expect to see as normal compensation.

If the CO_2 is up, but not as far as it should be, then it is partially compensated, and there may be a component of respiratory alkalosis involved.

Metabolic Acidosis:

If respiratory compensation for a metabolic acidosis is in place and behaving normally, then

Step 1: Multiple the bicarb value by 1.5,
Step 2: Add 8

The resulting number should equal the pCO_2. If it does not, there is a mixed disorder.

In reality, you don't really need steps 1 and 2. If you try the equation out (bicarb $\times 1.5 + 8$), it always turns out to be about the same as making a 1:1 correspondence between the *change in the bicarb,* and the change in the pCO_2. In other words, if the bicarb has dropped by about nine points compared to the normal value, then the pCO_2 should have decreased by about the same amount, nine points, if it is compensating properly.

Please note: The approximation described will only give you a good result if the pH is fairly near to the normal 7.4 value. If the patient's pH is very abnormal, the 1:1 relationship changes, eventually approaching 1:2!

Acid-Base Problems: "Just the Facts"

These guidelines represent a general approach to acid-base disorders and the data you will see for patients with acid-base disorders. More precise ways of calculating expected changes in these values are available. These methods are, however, significantly more difficult to recall and use in a pinch on an exam or in the hospital. Understand, though, that the values you will obtain are approximate.

The normal values listed below can, in fact, take on a range of normal values. For the sake of simplicity, memorize a single value, and know that values very close to it are likely to be normal.

Normal values that must be memorized:

Normal pH = 7.4   Normal pCO2 = 40   Normal HCO3- = 24

Acid-base disorders come in two possible flavors, acidemia (meaning unusually large amounts of acid in the bloodstream) **and alkalemia** (meaning unusually large amounts of base in the blood). These may result from **alterations in either the respiratory or the metabolic systems**. When either of these systems is "out of whack," **the other system will try to bring the pH back toward normal.** In other words, one system will "compensate" for the other system to the extent it can. This is what is meant by a "compensated acid-base disturbance." It means that an acid-base disturbance actually exists, but it might not be obvious initially because the other system has compensated returning the pH to normal (or near normal). The kidney is in charge of modifying the HCO3- balance.

Occasionally two acid-base disturbances exist in the same patient at once (for example, a respiratory alkalosis and a metabolic alkalosis – for example, a hyperventilating patient who has been vomiting a lot). This is called a mixed acid-base disorder. The rules below will help you to figure out when this is the case, although mixed disorders are inherently a little more confusing than the simple derangements.

Here are the basic guidelines for figuring out what kind of acid-base disturbance you've got, and whether the other system has been able to compensate for the problem or not.

Respiratory acidosis

If the pH goes down by 0.1 (to pH = 7.3), then the pCO2 should go up by 10 (pCO2 = 50) if it is purely respiratory.

Exception: If the respiratory acidosis is chronic, as in COPD, then the pH change is less (as you would expect) for each increase of 10 in the pCO2. The pH will drop about 0.03 for each change of 10 in the pCO2.

(Note: To make the estimate as accurate as possible, you can use 0.08 in cases of respiratory acidosis or alkalosis, rather 0.1. For example, this means that in respiratory acidosis, if the pH goes down by 0.08 (to pH = 7.32), then the pCO2 should go up by 10. If, however, you find acid-base relationships hard enough to remember in their simplest versions, just use 0.1 for all of them (respiratory & metabolic, acidosis & alkalosis). It will still give you a good idea of what you are dealing with.)

Respiratory alkalosis

If the pH goes up by 0.1 (pH = 7.5), then the pCO2 should go down by 10 (pCO2 = 30).

Metabolic acidosis

If the pH goes down by 0.1 (pH = 7.3), then the HCO3- should drop by about 10 (HCO3- = 14) if the acidosis is purely metabolic.

Metabolic alkalosis

If the pH goes up by 0.1 (pH = 7.5), then the HCO3- should increase by about 10 (HCO3- = 34 or a little less than that) if it is all metabolic.

Compensated acid-base disorders are cases in which the HCO3- or pCO2 is clearly abnormal, but the pH is normal or near normal. **There are limits** to how much HCO3- and pCO2 can correct the pH. The pCO2 compensation mechanism usually cannot provide a pCO2 greater than 55 (people just can't manage to breathe any less than that). Similarly, it is difficult to get a pCO2 to less than 12 mmHg because you would "tire out" from a respiratory standpoint to maintain such a low plasma CO2 level. The compensatory HCO3- response usually can't go higher than about 30 mEq/L in an acute situation because the kidneys don't "activate" their long-term strategy "ammonia-genesis" until after 2–3 days of persistent acidemia. For people with chronic acidosis, the kidney has more time to develop ways of delivering additional HCO3- to the body. In these patients, such as COPD patients, the HCO3- may reach 55 mEq/L (the same number as the pCO2 maximum).

How do you know when you have a mixed acid-base disorder on your hands? When you check for the simple correlations listed above and you do not find them, you probably have a mixed disorder. (These are the same relationships described in the text above.)

	pH	pCO2	HCO3-
Respiratory acidosis	↓0.1 (or 08)	↑10	↑ if compensating (changes the pH value)
Respiratory alkalosis	↑0.1 (or 08)	↓10	↓ if compensating (changes the pH value)
Metabolic acidosis	↓0.1	↓ if compensating	↓10
Metabolic alkalosis	↑0.1	↑ if compensating	↑10 (or a little less)

Suppose you have a patient with a metabolic acidosis. The respiratory system should try to compensate by decreasing the pCO2. If the pH has declined by approximately 0.1, then you expect the pCO2 to decline by about 10 mmHg as an attempt at compensation. If, however, the obtained pCO2 is actually decreased by only 5, then you have both metabolic acidosis and respiratory acidosis. (This assumes that the patient has been acidotic for a long enough period of time for compensation to work.)

On the other hand, suppose you have another patient with metabolic acidosis with the same laboratory numbers. For this patient, though, there is one difference. The pCO2 is decreased by 15 instead of the expected 10. In this case, your patient has a metabolic acidosis with a respiratory alkalosis.

Remember that the compensatory mechanisms for acid-base disturbances never "overcorrect" beyond the normal pH.

Chapter 6
General Nephrology Question and Answer Items

What is the other name for Berger's disease?	**IgA nephropathy**
What seems to be the trigger for Berger's disease?	**A viral infection** (mainly URIs with activation of mucosal defenses)
What is the usual long-term outcome in Berger's disease?	**Spontaneously resolves**
Which post-infectious nephropathy has low complement levels?	**Post-strep has low C3**
What do you see in the kidney of a post-strep nephritis patient?	**"Humps" on the basement membrane**
If a nephritis patient has sensorineural deafness and cataracts, what should you suspect is the cause?	**Alport syndrome**
What is the long-term outcome for Alport nephritis?	**Usually end-stage renal failure in teens or 20s**
If a patient has microscopic or gross hematuria and nephrolithiasis, what should you suspect?	**Idiopathic hypercalciuria (although the blood could be due to a stone that formed for another reason)**

© Springer Science+Business Media New York 2016
C.M. Houser, *Pediatric Tricky Topics, Volume 2*,
DOI 10.1007/978-1-4939-3109-5_6

What medication should you *avoid* in a hypercalciuria patient?	Furosemide (Lasix®) – it increases calcium excretion further
What medication is *helpful* for a hypercalciuria patient?	Thiazide diuretic (increases calcium retention)
What dietary modifications are helpful in hypercalciuria?	Decrease oxalate-containing foods (chocolate, nuts, tea) – *Do not decrease calcium-containing foods* (Decreasing high-salt foods is also helpful, because increased Na intake promotes increased calcium excretion)
Which kidney problem is associated with loss of "foot processes" on the glomerulus?	Minimal change disease
What accounts for 80 % of the nephrotic syndrome cases seen in children?	Minimal change disease
What is the triad of nephrotic syndrome?	Edema Proteinuria/low albumin Hyperlipidemia
What is the description of the typical minimal change disease patient?	Male aged 2–8 years
How is minimal change disease treated?	Steroids & cyclophosphamide, if needed
How is nephrotic syndrome treated, if the patient's condition requires it?	25 % albumin fluids & furosemide & Often steroids (it may also be necessary to tap the ascites, but usually not)

ACE inhibitors & angiotensin II receptor blockers are frequently used in patients with nephrotic syndrome. What are the two main purposes for using them?

To manage hypertension

&

Decrease proteinuria

What is the classic presentation for children with renal dysfunction?

Periorbital edema

Alport nephritis, hypercalciuria, IgA nephropathy, and post-infectious glomerulonephritis all commonly present with what finding?

Gross or microscopic hematuria

(post-infectious glomerulonephritis includes post-strep glomerulonephritis)

Which type(s) of RTA produces acidosis and a *urine* anion gap?

Type 4
(also causes hyperkalemia)

What is distal RTA?

Failure to excrete hydrogen

If there is metabolic acidosis, but no anion gap (normal anion gap, in other words), what are the likely causes?

Diarrhea or an RTA

Which RTA is characterized by severe bicarb wasting?

Proximal
(also known as RTA type 2)

If the kidney is wasting a lot of bicarb, what other problems develop?

Wasting of glucose, phosphate, and amino acids

Which type of RTA often accompanies congenital disorders and inborn errors of metabolism?

Proximal RTA
(also known as RTA type 2)

A low urine chloride (<10 mEq) suggests what possible underlying problems?

Gastric fluid losses
Diarrhea
Cystic fibrosis

A high urine chloride (>10 mEq) in a patient with high blood pressure suggests what two diagnoses?

Cushing's syndrome or
Hyperaldosteronism

If the urine chloride is high, and blood pressure is normal, what are the most likely causes?	**Acute diuretic use** **Bartter's syndrome**
Which psychiatric medication sometimes causes DI?	**Lithium**
Normal urine output for an infant?	**1–2 cc/kg/day**
How can you calculate an approximate "bladder capacity?" (in ounces)	**Child's age + 2** **For metric results use:** **7 × weight in kg = mL in infants** **Age in years × 30 + 30 = mL in children**
How is proteinuria diagnosed?	**Either a 24-h urine** *or* **A spot urine**
When can proteinuria be a normal finding?	**Alkaline urine** **Concentrated urine** (high specific gravity)
How does the urine protein/creatinine ratio help you diagnose proteinuria in kids?	**Urine protein/urine creatinine >0.2 diagnoses proteinuria** **(However, nephrotic range proteinuria is >2.0)**
How can you use the urine protein-creatinine ratio to diagnose proteinuria in an infant older than 6 months?	Same process, but >0.5 is considered proteinuria in infants (6–24 months)
Which aspects of history are especially important to pay attention to in renal questions?	**Edema** **UTI history** **Toxin exposure** **Hearing loss** (Hearing loss is associated with certain causes like Alport syndrome, or drug side effects, and is also a tip-off to possible renal dysfunction in newly presenting patients, because renal patients have an unusually high rate of sensorineural hearing loss)

If a question states that urine has both protein and bacteria in it, which is probably more important?	**The bacteria**
What is a common presenting complaint for hypercalciuria – *even if no kidney stones have formed?*	**Abdominal pain and dysuria**
What is the main underlying problem that leads to the nephrotic syndrome?	The glomerulus is too leaky (Podocyte dysfunction and loss of basement membrane negative charge are involved)
Patients with nephrotic syndrome appear to be fluid overloaded, because they are edematous. What is their main fluid or electrolyte issue?	Intravascular fluid depletion (It's all leaked out!)
What are the immune consequences of nephrotic syndrome?	**Poor immune function – IgG & complement are low (they leak out, also)**
What infection are nephrotic syndrome patients at special risk of developing?	**Encapsulated organisms (such as *Strep pneumo* and *H. flu*)**
If nephrotic syndrome patients have low intravascular fluid volume, why are they so edematous?	Low albumin means low oncotic pressure, so fluid leaks into the tissues
What special vascular complication are nephrotic syndrome patients at unusual risk to develop?	**Thrombosis of major vessels, especially the renal vein (due to loss of antithrombin III into the urine)**
Benign proteinuria is fairly common. 50 % of benign proteinuria patients have what etiology?	**Orthostatic proteinuria**
What is orthostatic proteinuria?	**Protein falls through the glomerulous when the patient stands up – (literally, more proteinuria with standing)**

How do you diagnose orthostatic proteinuria?

Compare protein amounts in morning urine versus urine later in the day

What are some common causes of (benign) transient proteinuria? (4)

1. Dehydration
2. Exercise (especially extended running or marching)
3. Fever
4. Minor trauma (like a minor MVC)

A healthy 8-year-old child is found to have proteinuria (without edema) when Mom brings him in for "frothy" urine. Nothing else is found on history or physical exam. What is the *next step* in management?

Repeat the UA with a morning urine 3× over the next several weeks – it is probably transient (without identifiable reason).

(Some sources recommend fewer checks, but up to four are recommended – persistent proteinuria is concerning but quite rare in kids)

What finding in the urine tells you that there is probably glomerular disease?

RBC casts

How is microscopic hematuria defined?

Five or more RBCs per high powered field in two fresh urine samples (centrifuged)

Which common pediatric hematological disorder causes hematuria fairly often?

Sickle cell

What sort of kidney damage is both common and painful, for sickle cell patients?

Papillary necrosis (of the kidney parenchyma)

How can muscle damage fool you into thinking there's a primary kidney problem?

UA *strip* will come up positive for blood – but it's actually reading the myoglobin, rather than hemoglobin

Should patients with microscopic hematuria have a cystoscopy?

Generally, no
(too invasive)

(The most common reason for the hematuria is benign familial thin basement membrane disease)

Will Berger's disease patients have high IgA in the serum?

Sometimes

In addition to Berger's disease, which other disorder has IgA complexes in the vessels (including the glomerulus)?

Henoch–Schonlein purpura

When is a patient most likely to develop hematuria due to Berger's disease?

Acute illnesses
(including minor ones such as URI)

Which causes of nephritis have low complement levels?
(3)

Lupus
Post-infectious
Membranoproliferative

Is it common to have relapses of minimal change disease?

Yes – especially in the first 3 years after diagnosis – usually goes away permanently by adolescence

What are the two main causes of dysuria?

Infection & local irritation/trauma

(vaginitis, ulcers, chemical or clothing irritation, poor hygiene)

What parasite is an unusual cause of dysuria in children?

Pinworms!

(much more common on boards than in your office!)

What is "diurnal enuresis?"

Child >3 years
Never been dry

(in particular, it refers to daytime involuntary wetting)

How is diurnal enuresis best treated?	Noninvasive treatments beginning with hydration & timed voiding, treatment of constipation (if needed), & in some cases pelvic floor exercises
	(Note: invasive treatment such as periodic straight cathing was used more in the past – not currently recommended unless other options fail or are not appropriate)
Is diurnal enuresis common?	**No**
	(by age 7 years, just 3 % of girls & 2 % of boys)
What are appropriate ways to help a child with nighttime enuresis get dry? (2 meds, 1 device, 1 strategy)	**Developmental (wait for child to outgrow wetting) Wetting alarms Desmopressin Imipramine (TCA)**
	(TCAs are less commonly used due to possible side effects)
What is the natural course of enuresis?	**Eventually goes away in adolescence, if not before**
What percentage of kids with nocturnal enuresis will spontaneously "get better" per year – with no treatment?	**15 %**
Can drinking too much water cause bedwetting?	Yes – especially just before bed, or in cases of polydipsia
A common cause of urinary difficulties, including enuresis, is related to the gut. What is it?	**Constipation/encopresis**
If a child has recurrent UTIs, and no anatomic explanation can be found on VCUG, how should the child be managed?	**Trial of prophylactic antibiotics** (care coordinated with urology)
If a urine culture grows <10,000 colonies, how should you interpret that?	**Not significant – usually a contaminant**

What is the magic number of colony forming units that means you can be confident of your urine culture results (if the sample was collected properly)?	**50,000 in children age 2–24 months (of a single microbe)** *Note: This is a change from 100,000!*
How many colony-forming units are needed to diagnose UTI in an infant less than 2 months old?	**10–50,000**
Which virus likes to cause UTIs?	**Adenovirus**
What is the most common bacterial cause of UTI?	*E. coli* **(Enterococcus, Proteus, & Klebsiella are more unusual causes)**
If a preschool child has a suspected first UTI, what is the correct work-up?	**Urinalysis & urine culture** **CBC & metabolic panel IF pyelonephritis suspected** **Blood cultures IF bacteremia or sepsis suspected** **Consider need for ultrasound (renal & bladder)**
Which first-time UTI patients do not require any imaging studies?	**Afebrile or rapid defervescence (<72 h after antibiotic started)** **Good follow-up** **Normal voiding pattern (not dribbling)** **No abdominal masses detected**
VCUGs (voiding cystourethrograms) are not done as often as they were in the past. According to current guidelines, when should you consider a VCUG for a UTI patient? **(2 situations)**	**After a second febrile UTI episode** **Or** **After a first febrile UTI with reason to suspect structural issues** (e.g., mass, obstruction, hydronephrosis, scarring)

Is the urinary nitrite test useful for diagnosing UTI in children?	Yes, when it is positive – but a negative result is inconclusive (not all microbes produce nitrite, and children usually void frequently, so the urine is often not in the bladder for the 4 h required to produce nitrite from dietary nitrate present in the urine)
Is urine collected in a bag attached to the perineum useful in diagnosing UTI?	Only to rule it out – Positive results CANNOT be used, regardless of technique
If you find asymptomatic bacteriuria on screening, what is appropriate follow-up?	Nothing to do
A "unilateral flank mass" is often due to what renal cause? (2)	Enlarged multicystic dysplastic kidney Or Hydronephrosis
How do you evaluate a child for possible vesicoureteral reflux (VUR)?	VCUG
Which children are most likely to have reflux as a cause of UTIs or other urological problems?	The youngest kids
Is the kidney damaged by ureteral reflux, if there are no infections or other complications?	Generally not – The damage results from infection, sterile reflux is usually okay
The chance of spontaneous VUR resolution is related to the child's age. What should you expect for children <1 year old?	Most cases spontaneously resolve (especially in boys)
What should you expect for the natural course of VUR found in a 1–5 year old child?	Grades I–III usually resolve Grades IV & V may resolve

Vesicoureteral reflux is "graded" with five grades. If a vignette says your patient has grade 1 or 2, what should you do?

Monitor with periodic cultures & monitor with yearly scans

Or

Treat with prophylactic antibiotics & monitor with yearly scans until hydronephrosis resolves

(optimal management remains an area of debate for low-grade reflux)

If the VCUG report indicates grades 4 or 5 reflux, what does that mean for management?

Urology referral – surgery could be required

What is the recommended initial management for grade 3 vesicoureteral reflux?

Prophylactic antibiotics

&

Yearly VCUG or RNC/DMSA to evaluate for resolution vs. worsening

(RNC = Radionuclide cystogram)

In what circumstances is grade III VUR often managed surgically?

Bilateral grade III VUR
Complicated by infection despite antibiotics
Persistent grade III VUR (over several years)

How do you know when your patient has glomerulonephritis?

HTN + hematuria + proteinuria = glomerulonephritis

What causes post-infectious glomerulonephritis?

Immune complex deposition in the kidney

Post-strep glomerulonephritis can occur after what type(s) of GABHS infections?

Throat or skin

How do the boards like to describe hematuria?

Tea- or cola-colored urine, sometimes "rusty" or "smoky"

Post-infectious glomerulonephritis can also have low serum albumin (like nephrotic syndrome). Why does this happen?

Hemodilution (not due to protein loss in urine)

What is the classic triad of post-strep glomerulonephritis?

Hematuria
Edema
Hypertension

Which two glomerulo-nephritides often lead to renal failure?

Focal segmental glomerulosclerosis

&

Membranoproliferative glomerulonephritis

Focal segmental glomerulosclerosis is usually seen in what age group?

Adolescents

What other findings indicate that a renal biopsy is a good idea? (4)

Hypertension
Low complement level (could be membranoproliferative)
Proteinuria
Decreased kidney function

How can you remember the three glomerulo-nephritides that lead to low complement levels?

If you had PMS, you wouldn't be in the mood for "compliments" ("complements")
P Post-infectious
M Membranoproliferative
S SLE (lupus)

How can you differentiate post-infectious glomerulonephritis serologically from the other two causes of low complement levels?

Complement C3 returns to normal after about 2 months in post-infectious
The ones with permanent kidney damage stay low

What is the triad of hemolytic uremic syndrome (HUS)?

Hemolytic anemia
Renal failure
Thrombocytopenia

Are serum complement levels low in HUS?

No

Will the Coombs test for anemia be positive or negative with HUS?	Negative

What history do HUS patients often present with?

Abdominal pain after eating bad cow-related items (meat or milk)

(also associated with exposure to apple juice/cider and water parks)

What symptoms do HUS patients most often present with?

Prodrome of low-grade fever & diarrhea – >80 % with obvious bloody diarrhea

Irritability & pallor

Abdominal pain & vomiting

What other findings often accompany HUS?

Skin & CNS changes

What is the classic bacteria associated with HUS?

E. coli 0157:H7

What new treatment for HUS should you be aware of?

Eculizumab – very effective, but very expensive

(used in "atypical HUS" which targets the kidney with thrombi, often causing renal failure)

If the history of a renal patient includes "prematurity," what should you think about?

Umbilical artery catheterization may have injured the renal artery

Why are patients with chronic renal failure pale?

Low level of erythropoietin, so the RBC count drops

If a patient with hypertension is described as having *muscle cramps or muscular weakness*, what etiology should you think of?

Hyperaldosteronism

(the hypokalemia is causing the muscle symptoms)

If the vignette describes flushing, palpitations, diarrhea, and fever, along with hypertension, what etiology should you think of?

Pheochromocytoma

If hypertension begins at the same time as sexual development, what is the likely etiology? (general category)

An enzyme deficiency in the adrenal glands

What electrolyte disturbances do you expect to see in chronic renal failure patients?

Hyperkalemia
Hypocalcemia/hyperphosphatemia
& Metabolic acidosis

What endocrine & growth issues do chronic renal failure patients have?

Hyperparathyroidism
& Failure to thrive

Do renal failure patients have immune issues?

Yes, their immune cells do not work as well as usual

Do renal failure patients have clotting issues?

Often yes – the platelets don't work as well as usual

(usually related to increased BUN level)

How is uremia managed in children with chronic renal failure?

Protein restriction mainly

When a vignette seems to be describing hypertension, what must you always remember to look for?

Wrong cuff size used

Or

BP not obtained manually
(machine readings may not always be reliable)

Which two enzyme deficiencies most often cause hypertension?

11-Hydroxylase deficiency &
17-Hydroxylase deficiency

What unusual problem is more likely in neonates who've received considerable amounts of furosemide? (For example, due to cardiac problems)

Nephrocalcinosis & renal stones

What proportion of posterior urethral valve (PUV) patients will eventually develop end stage renal disease?

About 1/3

Which aspects of PUV cause kidney damage?
 (3 main ones)

Abnormal pressure during kidney development causes renal dysplasia

Increased bladder pressures after birth

Recurrent UTIs are common

For patients born with a posterior urethral valve, what are the known risk factors for progression to renal failure?
                (3)

Elevated nadir creatinine of >1 mg/dL during the first year of life

Need for (chronic) catheterization

Bladder dysfunction with increased leak point pressure & poor wall compliance

Renal & genitourinary symptoms related to PUV often increase at what developmental period?

Puberty –
Increased metabolic demand on the kidney & developmental changes in the bladder

Why is it important to follow the GFR & serum BUN and creatinine over the first year of life, when assessing renal function?

Because the kidney continues its maturational process after birth –
Initial measurements may not accurately reflect the true level of renal function

Chapter 7
General Urology Question and Answer Items

Do hydroceles require treatment?

Generally, no
(unless they become very large)

Which scrotal masses transilluminate?

Hydroceles

    &

Spermatoceles

What is a spermatocele?

A fluid collection in the outbound ducts of the scrotum

How can you identify a spermatocele?

1. Transilluminates
2. Doesn't change with Valsalva
   (varicocele would)
   (hernia would)
3. Mass is behind & above testis

If something on the scrotal exam is described as being like a "bag of worms," what is the mass?

A varicocele
(dilated, tortuous veins)

What is a varicocele?

Dilated veins in the scrotum
(usually left sided)

Which veins are dilated in varicoceles?

The "pampiniform" plexus
(of the scrotum)

© Springer Science+Business Media New York 2016
C.M. Houser, *Pediatric Tricky Topics, Volume 2*,
DOI 10.1007/978-1-4939-3109-5_7

How do you identify a varicocele?	• **Usually left sided** • **"Bag of worms" consistency** • **Increased size with Valsalva** • **Decreases when lying down**
Does a varicocele require treatment?	If the testis becomes hypotrophic or if sperm count decreases – Yes (otherwise, no)
Is treatment needed for spermatoceles?	No
Do spermatoceles affect fertility?	No
What is a hematocele?	Blood in the scrotal sac due to trauma
Do hematoceles require treatment, and if so, what is it?	• **If they become very large, then yes** • **Surgical drainage**
How are hematocele symptoms treated?	**Pain meds** **Ice packs** **Scrotal elevation/bed rest**
If a testicular neoplasm develops, is it usually painful or painless?	**Painless**
Why might a testicular tumor patient present with back pain?	Retroperitoneal LAD (associated with tumor)
What percentage of testicular tumors develops from germ cells, as opposed to structural (stromal) tissue of the testis?	**95 %**
If infection affects the testis itself, what is it called?	**Orchitis**
If a testis atrophies following orchitis, what pathology is the patient at increased risk to develop?	Testicular cancer

Infertility following orchitis is usually accompanied by what physical exam finding?	Bilateral atrophy
If mumps produces orchitis, what is the treatment?	Supportive only
What are the most common causal organisms for epididymitis in an adolescent male?	1. *C. trachomatis* (most common) 2. *N. gonorrhoeae* (*E. coli* & pseudomonas are also occasional culprits)
How are the Doppler flow studies or radionucleotide scans different for epididymitis/orchitis vs. testicular torsion?	**Infection → increased flow & perfusion** **Torsion → decreased flow & perfusion**
Which two radiological modalities are most preferred for evaluation of the scrotal area?	US and MRI
Is "torsion of the spermatic cord" the same thing as "torsion testis?"	Yes
In a newborn male, how long should the penis be?	3–4 cm
At what penile length would an endocrine work-up definitely be indicated?	2.5 cm
Should the scrotum have rugae at the time of a full-term birth?	Yes
If one testicle has not descended, how will the scrotal findings at birth be different from usual?	Less rugae & Empty scrotal sac (on one side)
"Chordee," or a ventral curving penis, usually accompanies what minor penile malformation?	Hypospadias *(although chordee often occurs without hypospadias)*

What usually is the course
for hydroceles present at birth?

Slowly resolves spontaneously

True or false. The foreskin should
be retracted on newborns to permit
proper cleansing?

False –
It is often adherent & will be damaged
by retraction

At what age is it alright to fully
retract a foreskin?

Three years old

If genitalia are ambiguous,
and the newborn is otherwise doing
well, what is the first consultation/
testing type you should pursue?

Genetics –
Figure that out first
Then sort out the endocrine and
developmental issues

What is "epispadias?"

The meatal opening is on the top midline
of the penis
(vs. hypospadias, on the bottom)

Is torsion of the testicular
appendage painful?

Yes

Is torsion of the testicular
appendage a surgical emergency?

No –
No treatment needed other than pain
control

What is manual detorsion of a testis?

A usually *un*successful attempt to correct
torsion non-operatively

**If one testis is documented to be
in torsion, why would surgery be
recommended for both testes?**

**Increased probability of torsion means
both should be surgically fixed if one
torses**

**How does testicular torsion
present?**

**Unilateral groin pain/abdominal pain
with swelling of the affected testis**

+/− nausea/vomiting

What rather unreliable sign of
testicular torsion is often mentioned
on board exams?

Loss of cremasteric reflex
(testis doesn't move up when thigh is
stroked)

Generally, the pain of testicular
torsion should be sudden onset and
constant. Why could it also present as
intermittent pain?

Sometimes the testis spontaneously
detorses, and then torses again, creating
intermittent pain

Is a torsed testicle tender to palpation?	Yes
How is torsion of the appendix testis managed?	Supportive care – Pain meds & anti-inflammatories
Where is the appendix of the testis?	Upper pole (It is about the size of a pea)
What will a radionuclide scan, or Doppler flow study, show if the problem is torsion of the appendix testis?	**Normal or sometimes increased uptake/flow** (due to the inflammation)
What does "blue dot" sign refer to in urology?	**When the testicular appendage torses – You see a sharply defined blue area through the skin (small)**
What is the most common cause of testicular pain in boys 2–11 years old?	Torsion of the "appendix testis" (rare in older age groups)
What is Prehn's sign?	Decreased testicular pain with elevation of the testes
Pain that decreases with testicular elevation suggests what diagnosis?	**Epididymitis**
Will the cremasteric reflex be present or absent for patients with epididymitis?	**Present**
What is the typical age group for testicular torsion?	<30 years
What is the special term for the anatomical variation that leads to testicular torsion?	**"Bell clapper deformity"**
What is the most common cause of testicular pain in boys 12–18 years old?	Testicular torsion

If a patient with testicular torsion elevates a testicle what happen to his pain?	No change Or Worsening pain
Mumps orchitis can cause sterility, but usually does not. Why not?	It is frequently unilateral
What is the average age range for development of testicular cancer?	20–40 years
How is testicular torsion treated?	Emergency surgical fixation of *both testes*
What is the usual source of epididymitis in men less than 50 years old, and how is it treated?	• STDs • Ceftriaxone & doxycycline or azithromycin
Which testicular tumors may cause precocious puberty in males, and why?	• Leydig cell tumors • They secrete androgens
What is the most common type of testicular tumor?	Seminoma (a type of germ cell tumor)
What are the mainstays of treatment for testicular cancer? (2)	1 Orchiectomy 2 Radiation
What four findings suggest urethral injury?	**1. Boggy or "high-riding" prostate (depending on age)** **2. *Blood at the meatus*** **3. Severe pelvic fracture** **4. *Scrotal or perineal ecchymosis***
If one of the four signs of urethral injury is present, what must you not do until further diagnostics are completed, and what is the additional diagnostic needed?	• No Foley! • A retrograde cystourethrogram

What is the difference between an incarcerated hernia and a strangulated hernia?

- **Incarcerated hernias are stuck, but still have blood supply**
- **Strangulated bowel is stuck *and blood supply is compromised***

Does replacing a cryptorchid testicle in the scrotum change the probability of later testicular cancer?

No

(. . . and the higher it was, the greater the chance of cancer developing . . .)

When are undescended testes typically surgically moved to the scrotum?

At about 12 months

What are the main risks of leaving cryptorchid testes in place?
(3)

1. **Malignancy**
2. **Infertility**
3. **Torsion**

Which is preferred for cryptorchid testes, hormonal treatment or surgical relocation?

Surgical relocation

(hormones do stimulate testicular movement, but the success rate is not great)

What is the other name for a struvite renal stone?

Magnesium ammonium phosphate stone

What causes a struvite stone?

Ammonia-producing bacteria
(classically – proteus)

Struvite stones have a characteristic appearance. What is it?

"Stag horns"
(They fill the renal pelvices, so they look like antlers)

About 85 % of kidney stones can be seen on x-ray. Which ones cannot? (general type)

Uric acid stones

How are kidney stones usually treated?

<6 mm will pass on their own –

Give fluids
Pain control
Strainer to see what kind it was

What is special about uric acid stones?
(2)

1. Usually not seen on X-ray
2. May dissolve in alkaline urine!

If a stone will not pass,
how can it be removed?

Surgically
(endoscopically, if possible)

Or

Lithotripsy

How are kidney stones confirmed?

Renal ultrasound

Or

CT stone protocol

Most renal stones are made
of _____?

Calcium
(75 %)

Although most calcium stones
happen to otherwise healthy people,
what *conditions* put the patient
at increased risk?
(3)

Malignancy
Hyperparathyroidism
Small bowel bypass

What conditions increase
the patient's chance of developing
uric acid stones?
(2 groups)

• Gout
• Leukemia

(at time of treatment)

Will a CT of the kidney show
you whether a kidney stone
is causing your patient's pain?

No –
Symptomatic stones *are not in the
kidney,*
they are in the ureter, or at the UPJ
(ureteropelvic junction)

If a patient is found to have renal
stones while he or she is being
evaluated for something else,
what should you do?

Usually nothing –
Stones in the kidney are asymptomatic &
don't ordinarily cause problems

In otherwise healthy people, what
puts you at risk for kidney stones?
(2)

1. Dehydration
2. Personal or family history of stones

Should renal colic (kidney stone) patients be admitted?

Usually not –
Give fluids
Pain control
Antiemetics if needed
(Strainer to go home with)

If a stone does not pass while the patient is in the emergency department, can the patient still go home?

Yes –
If s/he can tolerate PO, can go home with pain meds

Which renal stone patients must be admitted?

1. **Pyelonephritis with stone**
2. **Uncontrollable pain**
3. **Uncontrollable vomiting**
4. **Single kidney**

(& sometimes hydronephrosis)

How long will it take a ureteral obstruction to damage the kidney if it causes hydronephrosis?

About *2 weeks!*

Which mumps complication affects the GU system?

Orchitis –
Can cause sterility
(but usually doesn't because it is typically unilateral)

Which patients develop acute urinary retention?
(2)

1. Benign prostatic hypertrophy (not usually seen in kids!)
2. Post-op or instrumented patients with clots

Why is it important to check for urethral injury in a trauma patient?

They will receive a Foley –
It's contraindicated if the urethra is injured!

If urethral injury is suspected, how do you evaluate it?

Retrograde cystourethrogram

(Put dye into the urethra, then check on X-ray to see whether it extravasates)

How are urethral disruptions (traumatic injuries) treated?

Sometimes surgically, Sometimes urology can place a tube to align the two parts, & let them heal

Why are varicoceles important?	They sometimes cause pain or infertility
How is a varicocele different clinically from a hydrocele?	• Hydroceles transilluminate • Varicoceles disappear if the patient lies down
How are varicoceles treated?	They are surgically resected (<u>if</u> symptomatic)
What treatment is needed for hydroceles?	Usually none
What *is* a hydrocele?	A collection of peritoneal fluid in the scrotum
What is peritoneal fluid doing in the scrotum?	It travels there through a slightly open processus vaginalis (processus vaginalis – the connective tissue sheath the testes migrate through to get to the scrotum)
What is hypospadias?	**Urethral meatus is on the bottom (ventral side) of the penis**
What critical item must you remember at the birth of a child with hypospadias?	**No circumcision –** **The foreskin may be needed for correction**
Is circumcision medically indicated?	**No –** **Unless the child has hydronephrosis/ reflux** (due to increased risk of UTIs in this population)
Are UTIs more common in uncircumcised males?	Yes – But still uncommon
What is phimosis?	When the foreskin is too tight on the glans to retract (for whatever reason – not necessarily a problem)

What is paraphimosis?

When the foreskin is retracted behind the coronal sulcus, and gets stuck!

What is the usual management for either phimosis or paraphimosis?

- **Manual reduction if possible**
- **Surgery often necessary (also to prevent recurrence)**

Why do posterior urethral valves only form in males?

In females, the structure becomes the hymen (so it is not incorporated into the bladder at all!)

Currently, when are most patients with posterior urethral valves diagnosed?

Before birth (via ultrasound)

If a patient is known to have a posterior urethral valve, what is the first & most important treatment goal?

Relief of the obstruction –
The valve must be removed as soon as possible, usually in the first few days after birth

After clearance of a posterior urethral valve, which study should be done to confirm that the valve is gone & the urethra appropriately healed?
(2)

VCUG

Or

Cystoscopy

(typically 1–3 months after the initial procedure)

If the valve (PUV) is removed shortly after birth, why do these patients often continue to have renal & GU difficulties?

Because the valve forms early in embryological/fetal development, so increased pressure in the upper tract (bladder & kidneys) was present during development & has already had an effect

In addition to renal changes occurring during development due to PUV, what other factors often contribute to decreased kidney function?

Elevated bladder pressures

&

Recurrent UTIs

If a PUV patient develops symptoms of urinary outlet obstruction, what complication should you especially consider?

Urethral stricture
(at or near the site of valve)

How commonly do PUV patients develop actual renal failure (end-stage renal disease)?	About 1/3
How common is diurnal enuresis in older (>5 years old) children with PUV?	About 1/3 – Usually related to elevated bladder storage pressure & poor emptying
What are the typical treatment options for enuresis in the older PUV patient? (3)	Anticholinergic medication Intermittent catheterization Bladder augmentation (usually with other tissues)
How long is follow-up needed for a patient who has had PUV as an infant?	Lifelong
How common is vesicoureteral reflux in patients with PUV?	Common – Present in up to 1/3 of patients (but thought to be due to abnormally high pressure, rather than an abnormal ureter insertion location)
What is vesicoureteral reflux dysplasia (VURD) syndrome?	A variation of PUV with vesicoureteral reflux mainly on one side, producing one hydronephrotic & nonfunctional kidney
Is VURD syndrome a good thing in a PUV patient?	No – Their risk of renal failure is the same as in PUV patients without VURD *(Note: This is a change – VURD syndrome was previously thought to be helpful, by allowing a sort of "pop-off" for the high pressures in the system to the dysfunctional kidney. Recent data has not shown this to be true)*
While PUV is not kind to the renal system, what is the more immediate threat to survival of the infant with PUV?	Pulmonary problems – Poor pulmonary development due to oligohydramnios (from the urinary outflow obstruction)

Which patients should automatically be evaluated for possible PUV shortly after birth?

Males with evidence of hydronephrosis on prenatal ultrasound

How is the evaluation for PUV generally done?

VCUG

Some PUV patients are not detected before or near the time of birth. For these late presentations, what symptoms are common?

UTI

Diurnal enuresis (also secondary) older than 5 years

Voiding difficulties, pain, or abnormal urinary stream

Which findings are suggestive of PUV, and which are definitive?

Suggestive:
Thickened or trabeculated bladder
Dilated or elongated urethra

If a patient with PUV has completed urodynamic studies early in childhood, and symptoms have not changed, is it necessary to repeat the studies later?

Yes –
Bladder compliance sometimes deteriorates over time

What are the consequences of the fibrotic & noncompliant bladder that can develop in PUV patients?
(4)

Increased risk for:
Urinary incontinence
Recurrent UTIs
Hydroureteronephrosis &
Renal function deterioration

(The bladder changes of significant noncompliance & fibrosis are sometimes known as "valve bladder")

During cystoscopy for correction of a PUV, what two complications involving the urethra are of special concern?

Urethral stricture
(possibly due to trauma during the procedure)

&

Urethral sphincter injury

How common is it for a second valve incision to be needed, after an apparently successful first one?

Common – about 1/3

(this is why a follow-up cystoscopy is often recommended as a routine measure 1–3 months after the initial procedure)

Chapter 8
General Dermatology Question and Answer Items

How can you remember which types of cells are found in scrapings from erythema toxicum neonatorum vs. transient neonatal pustular melanosis?

Erythema toxicum neonatorum = <u>E</u>os

<u>N</u>eonatal pustular <u>m</u>elanosis = <u>PMN</u>s

If an older child has a rash that looks like what you see in erythema toxicum neonatorum, what would you probably think it was?

Flea bites (helps you remember the appearance)

Is it possible to miss the vesicle phase of transient neonatal pustular melanosis, even if you have been examining the child from birth?

Yes – sometimes the disorder starts *in utero(!)* so the vesicle phase is already over when the baby is born

How often does aplasia cutis congenita occur as a single lesion?

70 %

Aplasia cutis congenita can occur anywhere on the body. Where are the lesions most often found?

80 % are scalp lesions – usually at the vertex (highest point on the scalp)

If you identify a lesion of aplasia cutis congenita, how should you treat it?

Usually heals on its own

© Springer Science+Business Media New York 2016
C.M. Houser, *Pediatric Tricky Topics, Volume 2*,
DOI 10.1007/978-1-4939-3109-5_8

If a lesion of aplasia cutis congenita has already healed on its own, how might you still notice on physical exam that the lesion was previously there?	No hair in a spot on the scalp – The lesion is deep enough that, even when it heals, there are no skin appendages present (glands, hair follicles, and hair)
If you see lesions on the extremities that look like cigarette burns, what infectious agent could be the culprit?	Crusted impetigo – due to GABS or staph
What are the only effective topical agents for impetigo?	Mupirocin (low cost, and good for limited disease), OR Retapamulin (newer agent)
Why might you want to culture impetigo?	Increasing incidence of MRSA
What is usually the best choice for treating impetigo, if an oral agent will be used?	Oral cephalexin
Do you need to worry about your patient developing rheumatic fever (or PANDAS – the neuropsych complications of strep infection), if he or she has developed impetigo?	No – skin infections don't do that (throat infections do) *(but post-strep glomerulonephritis is still possible)*
After infection with HHV-6, how long will the patient excrete the virus?	Lifetime – it's one of the herpes family! *(HHV-6 causes roseola)*
In which patients is the rash of roseola sometimes difficult to detect?	Dark skinned
If HHV-6 infection occurs in an immunocompromised host, the infection can be severe. What treatment is available?	Ganciclovir
What organism is associated with neonatal acne-like pustulosis (also called neonatal cephalic pustulosis)?	**Malassezia**
Neonatal acne-like pustulosis is clinically different from neonatal acne in what main aspect?	**No comedones**

At what point in life do port-wine stains become nodular and hypertrophied?

20s–40s

Pulsed-dye laser treatment is a good way to treat port-wine stains, although multiple treatments are usually required. When should laser treatment of port-wine stains ideally be attempted?

Before school age – To minimize psychosocial impact

(and definitely before the lesions worsen in adulthood)

If you treat a port-wine stain with pulsed dye laser, what must you warn the patient & family about?

They sometimes recur

What is the new name for a cavernous hemangioma?

"Deep" infantile hemangioma

("cavernous hemangioma" is no longer used in most literature)

There are two older terms for superficial infantile hemangioma. What are they?

Capillary hemangioma

&

Strawberry hemangioma

In general, are significantly sized hemangiomas of the genitals treated?

Yes – for both cosmetic and functional reasons

When hemangiomas occur in internal organs, which organs are most often affected?
(top 3)

1. Liver
2. GI
3. Brain
(in that order)

Avoiding which foods is usually a good idea for children with atopic dermatitis?

Cow's milk
Eggs
Wheat
Nuts

Can psoriasis have pustules?

Yes – there is a special type that has a lot of crusting and pus (called pustular psoriasis)

What is the most common systemic complication of psoriasis?

Psoriatic arthritis

After a herald patch appears, how long do you expect it to be before the whole rash of pityriasis rosea arrives?

A few days to a few weeks (not more than 2 weeks)

Which age group usually develops pityriasis rosea?	Adolescent/young adult
How often do patients with pityriasis have a recurrence after the first episode has cleared?	Rare
How long does the rash of pityriasis last?	1–2 *months!* (Let's hope it's not the type that itches!)
There are several types of ichthyosis. The most common one is ichthyosis vulgaris. Which part of the skin is spared in ichthyosis vulgaris?	The flexures
What is the course of ichthyosis vulgaris, as related to age?	**Appears after 3 months old,** & *improves with age*
How is X-linked ichthyosis different from ichthyosis vulgaris, in terms of its course?	Appears *before* 3 months old, & *worsens with age* (No, it doesn't worsen with sex!)
X-linked ichthyosis has several effects on other organs. Which problem is seen in both affected males and carrier females?	**Corneal opacities**
Males affected by **X-linked ichthyosis** often have what other (minor) congenital anomaly?	Cryptorchidism
What are the two types of contact dermatitis?	**Irritant & allergic**
How are the two types of contact dermatitis different?	Allergic requires previous exposure, and only certain people will develop it Irritant <u>does not</u> require prior exposure, and affects everyone exposed
Which medication causes *allergic* contact dermatitis most often?	Neomycin (topical ointment)

If a patient has been exposed to poison ivy, or something similar (an urushiol), can the dermatitis be spread by the fluid from the bers?	No
Can the contact dermatitis of poison ivy be spread by itching the area, then touching another area?	Sometimes – if the exposure was recent, the fat-soluble urushiol will still be in or on the skin – itching can lodge some under the nails and allow spread to another site
When treating a skin staph aureus infection how concerned should you be that it may not be sensitive to erythromycin?	Very – at least 1/3 are not
Which organism usually causes perianal cellulitis?	**Group A streptococcus**
What are the symptoms in kids with perianal cellulitis?	Perianal irritation & persistent red rash
How is perianal cellulitis usually treated?	**Systemic antibiotics (PCN or erythromycin)**
Perianal cellulitis is often misdiagnosed as what two other common problems?	Candidiasis or Perianal fissure
What clinical clue can point you to a diagnosis of staph scalded skin syndrome?	**Young child who doesn't want to be held (skin is very tender)**
We always hear about the sunburn-like rash and hypotension of toxic shock syndrome. Are other body systems also involved?	Yes, definitely (renal, hepatic, thrombocytopenia, CNS)
What is the special name for herpes infection/recurrence in unusual locations, sometimes experienced by wrestlers?	Herpes gladiatorum

For oral herpes lesions, which over-the-counter medication has good efficacy when applied every 3 h?

Docosanol
(trade name Abreva™)

Can herpetic whitlow sometimes appear to be a much bigger infection?

Yes – there are often swollen joints nearby, and sometimes red streaks/lymphangitis

Are chicken pox patients infectious <u>before</u> they get the rash?

Yes – at least 1 day before the rash

If a patient has been immunized for varicella, can he or she still get a zoster eruption (shingles)?

Yes – the live virus in the vaccine can cause it

Is zoster ber fluid infectious?

Yes – will cause chicken pox in vulnerable patients

If a patient has the rash of erythema infectiosum, and it seems to come and go, is the infection still likely to be erythema infectiosum?

Yes, the rash often comes & goes

If your patient has something that looks a lot like hand-foot-mouth disease, but there is <u>no mouth involvement</u>, what is it?

Papular – pruritic gloves and socks syndrome

Which virus typically causes "papular-pruritic gloves & socks syndrome?"

Parvovirus B19
(also seen with Coxsackie viruses, and some others)

Why are preemies at special risk for skin troubles?

Their skin is structurally different – The stratum corneum is *not* mature

What is the importance of the stratum corneum, and what is it?

- It is the topmost, tough layer of the skin
- Creates a barrier between us & outside!

When, in terms of gestational age, does the stratum corneum mature?

About 33 weeks

What is the easiest way to remember what the impact of immature skin will be for the preemie?
(Mnemonic & 5 consequences)

Mnemonic: Think of them like a burn patient

1. Lose heat
2. Lose fluids
3. Lose energy
4. Increased infection rate
5. Increased med absorption
   for topical meds

What very unusual cutaneous disease are preemies at special risk to develop?

Invasive (& then disseminated) fungal disease

In addition to preemies, what other patient group develops invasive fungal skin infections?

Severely immunocompromised (especially T cell dysfunction)

How do you identify invasive cutaneous fungal infections?

Well-defined "punched-out" appearance

Or

Black eschar

(in some cases, they may be more subtle, with subcutaneous nodules and plaques, but these presentations would usually require a specia's assistance to diagnose)

Which two fungi are especially likely to cause invasive cutaneous disease, in general?

Aspergillus

&

Rhizopus

Amongst premature and low-birth-weight infants, in particular, what fungi cause invasive cutaneous disease?

Candida
Aspergillus &
Less commonly Trichosporon and Curvularia

When should you suspect a cutaneous fungal infection in a preemie?

Anytime there is an ulceration (of the skin)

What causes the "miliaria" sometimes seen on the skin of infants & young children?

Obstruction of the sweat duct – eccrine gland

(usually by moist stratum corneum cells)

What is miliaria crystallina vs. rubra?

- Crystallina is very superficial obstruction, & causes only tiny vesicles
- Rubra is a little deeper, & causes 1–3 mm slightly red papules

If a child develops a rash in a hot environment, but *appears to be well*, and the contents of the papules/ papulopustules show *neutrophils but no bacteria*, what have you got?

Miliaria rubra

Where can miliaria rubra occur?

Almost anywhere – Including dorsal hands

(not on palms or soles, though)

If you are considering a diagnosis of miliaria rubra for a young child, what test should you do?

KOH prep to rule out candidiasis

(can look very similar)

A 2-day-old infant born at term develops blotches of red on the skin with overlying pustules. The infant is well appearing. What will a Wright stain of the pustule likely show, and what is the disorder?

- **Eosinophils and nothing else**
- **Erythema toxicum**

What is the natural course of erythema toxicum?

Spontaneous resolution by age 1 week

How do you recognize eosinophils on micro?

Bright red granules

       &

"Bilobed" nuclei

Which babies are most likely to develop erythema toxicum?

Term babies – Preemies almost never do

What is the difference between infantile & neonatal acne? **(2)**	**1. Time of development (neonatal is in first month)** **2. Infantile has comedones, neonatal does not**
How does neonatal acne present?	Small papules & pustules in the first month of life
What is the natural course of neonatal acne?	Spontaneously resolves in a few weeks or less
Should neonatal acne be treated?	No – Wait for resolution
Why does neonatal acne occur?	Androgen stimulation of sebaceous glands (etiology of infantile unclear)
What types of skin problems are seen with infantile acne?	Papules/pustules Comedones (open & closed) Nodules sometimes
What are the common terms for open & closed comedones?	Open = "Black head" Closed = "White head"
What is the usual course of infantile acne?	Spontaneous resolution after months – median time is about 18 months
Should infantile acne be treated?	If there are nodules – yes (risk of scarring)
When infantile acne is treated, how is it treated?	Retinoids (topical) Benzoyl peroxide Erythromycin (oral or topical)
Which ethnic groups commonly have "Mongolian spots?"	Asian African-American Native American
Where are Mongolian spots usually found?	Lower back & buttocks (they fade in time)

What is the new name for Mongolian spots?

Dermal melanocytosis

Transient neonatal pustular melanosis refers to what infant dermatological problem?

Superficial pustules →
Superficial erosions →
Hyperpigmented macules

(Hence, the name melanosis!)

How can you differentiate erythema toxicum from transient neonatal pustular melanosis, clinically?

1. **E. toxicum has pustules on a reddened macule – melanosis just has pustules**
2. **E. toxicum doesn't hyperpigment!**

How can you differentiate erythema toxicum from transient neonatal pustular melanosis, in terms of the lab findings?

- **Pustule scrapings of E. toxicum → eosinophils**
- **Pustule scrapings of melanosis → neutrophils**

(neither one should have any bacteria or fungus)

Which stage of transient neonatal pustular melanosis are you most likely to see, and why?

The hyperpigmented macules –

The pustules rupture very easily, so you often don't see them,
The hyperpigmentation lasts for months

What is the most common area of the body for bullous impetigo in infants?

Diaper area

What does bullous impetigo look like?

Large bers (bullae) –
One or more

Or

Superficial ulcer with collarette if they've ruptured

How can you identify ringworm infection?

- Growing border
- Well demarcated
- Central clearing

Does ringworm infection have pustules?

Not usually,
but it can

How can you tell the difference between a tinea infection (ringworm), and nummular eczema (eczema that occur in round, multiple, patches)?

Eczema is itchier

&

Has more dry skin

If a child has many spots of ringworm, what does that tell you about how he or she acquired the infection?

Usually came from a pet if it's that bad

Which patients are at increased risk of ringworm infection, although their immune systems are essentially normal?

Atopic patients

Clustered vesicles on an erythematous base is usually what skin infection?

Herpes simplex

If you see clustered vesicles on an erythematous base on a neonate, but you aren't certain of the diagnosis, what should you do?
   (3 things)

Send serology (IgM for HSV)
Send a viral culture (from the site)
Start empiric IV acyclovir

What is the other name for subcutaneous fat necrosis?

Panniculitis

(Remember that a pile of fat or fat roll is called a "pannus")

(but other forms of panniculitis also exist, such as those associated with lupus, erythema nodosum, etc.)

Which infants are at special risk of developing subcutaneous fat necrosis?
   (3 groups)

Those with:
1. Trauma
(including birth trauma)
2. Perinatal asphyxia
3. Hypothermia

What do subcutaneous fat necrosis areas look like on physical exam?

Ill-defined, erythematous plaques, indurated

(Can feel them better than you can see them)

Where is panniculitis most common in young infants?
   (4 areas)

Back
Buttocks
Legs
Cheeks

Where is panniculitis most common in older children?	Cheeks – Due to cold exposure (including popsicles!)
What is the course for panniculitis?	Spontaneous resolution
For a young infant, or a child with large amounts of panniculitis, what life-threatening complication sometimes develops?	Hypercalcemia! (Significant & life-threatening levels can be seen!)
What is neonatal lupus erythematosus?	**Development of some aspects of SLE in a newborn *due to transfer of maternal autoantibodies***
What proportion of mothers who have neonatal lupus erythematosus babies have a history of lupus, themselves?	½ (!) (Don't assume the Mom has to have a history!)
What is the prognosis for the *mother* if her baby has neonatal lupus, and she has no symptoms?	Increased risk of developing lupus – But not a certainty
How does neonatal lupus present, in general terms?	70 % skin findings *65 % cardiac* >50 % hepatobiliary
What are the usual skin findings of neonatal lupus?	• Usually, erythematous scaly lesions – can be widespread but most often seen on the scalp and face (can be worsened by sun exposure) • Most prominent around eyes (can be hypopigmented, also)
What is the usual course for neonatal lupus erythematosus?	Spontaneous resolution of skin lesions by 6 months (as maternal antibodies disappear) *(liver & hematological abnormalities also resolve spontaneously – heart block, if present, is permanent)*

If a neonate presents in third-degree heart block, what is the most common cause for the problem?

NLE
(Neonatal lupus erythematosus)

Third degree means no relationship between atrial and ventricular beats

Do neonatal lupus patients typically have other systems involved – aside from heart & skin?

No –
But 10–20 % have (cholestatic) hepatitis & thrombocytopenia

As neonatal lupus babies get a little older, what do you often find on the skin, in addition to the raccoon eye rash?

Annular scaly lesions
(annular = coin shaped)

What is the single best test to diagnose neonatal lupus erythematosus?

"Ro" antibody –
Test Mom & baby

(It is almost always positive in NLE)

What does a "collodion baby" look like?

Like the baby has an outer wrapping of kind of tight parchment

Although some collodion babies go on to have normal skin, most have what general category of underlying skin disorder?

Ichthyosis

Or

"Ichthyosiform" erythroderma

Because the outer surface of the skin is unusually tight, collodion babies are at risk to develop what problems at the eyes & mouth?

Eversion of eyelids & lips
(due to tension)

(In the eyelid, this is called "ectropion," while on the lips it is called "eclabium")

Aside from problems with eyes or mouth, collodion babies are also at risk for what other problems?

Same as a preemie –
The skin barrier is not intact (infection, fluid & heat loss, increased energy requirement)

Infants who have an impaired or missing stratum corneum (preemies, collodion babies, etc.) need what three interventions?

1. High humidity
2. Bland emollients (e.g., petroleum jelly)
3. Fluid/electrolyte monitoring

Infants with impaired strata corneum are most likely to develop what electrolyte problem?	Hypernatremia (due to dehydration)
Collodion babies are at special risk from what medication-related issue?	Increased absorption (especially of urea & acid-based agents sometimes used to improve their skin)
What is a "blueberry muffin" baby?	A baby with dark, raised spots on the skin – Due to extramedullary hematopoiesis
Where in the skin is the extramedullary hematopoiesis happening, for blueberry muffin babies?	**In the dermis**
There are a number of reasons for blueberry muffin babies – what is the most common?	**Congenital CMV**
What is the general idea behind blueberry muffin babies – in other words, what is the cause in general terms?	1. Anything that drops the crit low enough during fetal life can cause blueberry muffin baby 2. Viruses
In addition to CMV, give examples of other infectious diseases that might cause blueberry muffin babies. (3)	1. Rubella 2. Parvovirus B19 3. Coxsackie
What are some examples of low hemtocrit situations that might produce blueberry muffin baby? (4 important examples)	1. Twin-twin transfusion (for the losing twin) 2. Congenital leukemia 3. Blood grp/Rh incompatibility 4. Marrow infiltrating cancers
What does a baby with neonatal erythroderma look like?	Red, scaly baby
Is neonatal erythroderma a worrisome condition?	Yes – It's not difficult to manage, but often indicates other significant disorders are present

Erythroderma usually results from what three possible problems?
(3 groups)

1. **Infection (candida or staph scalded skin)**
2. **Immunodeficiency (SCIDs, GVH, etc.)**
3. **Ichthyosiform disorders**

A skin defect on the head is often an isolated defect, although it is also associated with trisomy 13. What characteristics should make you worry that the defect communicates *inside* the skull?

- It is midline
- It has a "hair collar" around it

What is a dermoid cyst of the skin?

A congenital tumor in the subQ tissue –
with dermal & epidermal type cells

Where do dermoid cysts of the skin usually develop?

Embryonic fusion lines

(especially the anterior fontanelle, upper lateral forehead, & submental area)

Submental = under the chin

Which dermoid cysts of the skin are most likely to produce complications?

Those with sinus tracts connecting them to the surface

(tuft of hair sometimes at surface)
(main complication is infection)

What is the recommended management for dermoid cysts?

Elective excision
(they sometimes turn malignant!)

A scalp nodule in the midline, present at birth, suggests _____?

Cranial dysraphism

(meaning underlying lack of closure with possible neural abnormalities)

Do dermoid cysts of the face or scalp frequently have intracranial connections?

No – only if they are midline (25 %)

What does a "hair collar" look like?

Dark, coarse, & longer hair surrounding a current or healed defect (suggests cranial dysraphism)

When is ultrasound a good way
to screen for spinal dysraphism?

- Infants <6 months
- Low level of suspicion

If ultrasound is *not* appropriate, what
diagnostic should you use to evaluate for
spinal dysraphism?

MRI

If an infant has spinal dysraphism, what
do you expect to find on physical exam?

Usually nothing
(can be lower extremity/anal perineal
findings, sometimes)

If the gluteal cleft deviates from midline
significantly, what is that likely to
indicate?

Underlying dysraphism

What type of vascular changes often
signal underlying dysraphism?

Hemangiomas & vascular stains
(= darkened areas of skin due to
dense capillary areas)

Spinal dysraphism typically occurs in
what portion of the spine?

Lower midline

Technically, are hemangiomas
malformations or tumors?

Tumors

What is the most common tumor of
infancy?

Hemangiomas

If a child has a hemangioma, will it be
present at birth?

Sometimes –
but they can appear up to 1–2 months
after birth

Which infants are *most likely* to have
hemangiomas?
   (3 risk factors)

Preemie girls with h/o chorionic
villus sampling

How common are hemangiomas in
1-year-old children?

10 %!

*(Data for 1-year-olds based on
Caucasian infants, due to lack of
data for other ethnicities. Percentage
with hemangiomas at birth is 1–2 %
in various ethnicities)*

Infantile hemangiomas come in two flavors – what are they?

Superficial & deep

("combined" is also a possibility)

How can you identify a superficial hemangioma?

Very red
Very well defined

(+ superficial is most common, so if in doubt, guess superficial!)

How does a deep hemangioma look different from a superficial hemangioma?

Deep are:
1. Either skin colored or violaceous
2. Raised
3. *Not* well defined

If a hemangioma is "mixed" or "combined" (same thing), what will it look like?

Ill-defined raised area

+

Some deep-red sharply demarcated areas

What is the most important complication to develop from liver hemangiomas?

High-output CHF!!!

Hemangiomas follow a characteristic pattern of growth, and they can be identified by it. What is the pattern?

**Proliferation
(weeks up to about a year)**

Stability

**Involution
(starts around 1 year, and takes years to finish)**

What is the first sign of involution for a superficial hemangioma?

Loss of the bright color –

**First central,
then peripheral**

Do deep hemangiomas involute faster or slower than the superficial ones?

Slower
(they soften & flatten)

After involution, does a hemangioma completely disappear, or does it leave residual changes?

Either –
Often some residual changes such as surplus skin or fibrofatty changes in the area

By age 5, what percentage of hemangiomas have involuted?	**>50 %** **(50 at 5)**
By age 9, what percentage of hemangiomas have involuted?	**90 %** **(90 at 9)**
Is bleeding from a hemangioma life threatening?	No – *(although it can still be pretty annoying!)*
A relatively common complication of hemangioma occurs mainly when the tumor is on the lip, nose, or perineum. What is the complication?	**Ulceration**
Which hemangiomas are most likely to ulcerate, in terms of their growth pattern?	Large & rapidly growing
What are the main concerns when a hemangioma ulcerates?	**Infection** **Scarring** **Bleeding** & **Pain**
How are hemangioma ulcerations managed?	• Vaseline or zinc oxide barrier protection • Occlusive dressing • Culture & antibiotics as needed
What are the main signs of infection in an ulcerated hemangioma?	Poor healing, or exudates (of course!)
What unrelated problem can look similar to a nasal hemangioma?	Encephalocele! (yikes!)
The bluish hue and raised nature of the dacryocystocele can look similar to which type of hemangioma?	Deep hemangioma (dacryocystoceles are accumulations between the eye & nose, related to the tear duct)

Why should an infant with a periorbital hemangioma have close monitoring from ophthalmology?
(2 reasons)

1. Possible obstruction of the visual axis and development of astigmatism
2. May have retroorbital hemangioma that you can't see (proliferative phase can be a big deal!)

Why might hemangiomas near the mouth, or on the neck, be concerning? (especially if bilateral)

Possibility of airway compromise (from subglottic hemangioma)

When hemangiomas are in very dangerous locations, or creating very serious complications, what is usually done to manage them?
(2 options)

Glucocorticoids or propranolol

(Propranolol appears to decrease hemangioma growth, as well as constrict the existing vessels)

How common are ocular complications with periorbital hemangiomas?

Very common – 80 %

How might a retroorbital hemangioma present on exam?

Proptosis

How are the steroids delivered when they are used to treat a problematic hemangioma?

Intralesional and/or systemic, depending on the lesion

What is the special name for hemangiomas that develop near the airway (chin, mandible, and upper neck)?

"Beard" hemangiomas

How do beard hemangiomas present, if they are threatening the airway?

The usual ways (Stridor, cough, hoarseness, noisy breathing, cyanosis)

If a baby presents to your practice at age 15 months with a beard hemangioma, how urgently should you be concerned about the airway?

Not concerned – The proliferative phase is over

What percentage of kids with extensive beard hemangiomas (4 out of 5 beard regions involved) will have airway involvement?

60 %

Lumbosacral hemangiomas are highly associated with disorder of what nearby structure?

Spinal cord – Tethered cord

What are the main complications of ear hemangiomas?

Disfiguring

&

Speech delay due to obstruction of the EAM

Lumbosacral hemangiomas are significantly associated with anomalies of what somewhat distant structure?

Kidneys

Is the dark skin of a port-wine stain a hemangioma?

No –
It is an area of permanent capillary malformation

Any idea what a "segmental cervicofacial" hemangioma is?

A large facial hemangioma that seems to follow an anatomic territory, such as the upper face

Why is it important to know about segmental cervicofacial hemangiomas?

Because they are part of the PHACES syndrome

What are the components of PHACES syndrome?

_P_osterior fossa malformations
   (like Dandy-Walker)
_H_emangioma
_A_rterial anomalies
   (intracerebral)
_C_ardiac anomalies/Coarc
_E_ye abnormalities
_S_ternal defects

If an infant has five cutaneous hemangiomas, what should you consider? (Or more than five, of course!)

"Diffuse neonatal hemangiomatosis"

(means that hemangiomas may be found in the organs)

Which organs are typically involved in cases of diffuse hemangiomatosis?

Liver (most common)
GI
CNS & eye

When hemangiomas occur in the liver, what special consequences can occur?

Portal hypertension & obstructive jaundice
(both are rare)

Patients with diffuse hemangiomatosis are at increased risk for what very important complication of hemangioma disease?

Congestive
 Heart
  Failure

What examinations should be considered for an infant with five or more cutaneous hemangiomas – in addition to a good physical exam?
(4)

1. Liver ultrasound (required)
2. Chest imaging
3. Check stool & urine for blood
4. Eye exam

How useful is laser therapy for hemangiomas?

Medium –
Lasers only penetrate about 1 mm, so it depends on the hemangioma

What is the main management approach to hemangioma?

"Active nonintervention"

(meaning parental guidance & monitoring of the lesion)

When medical intervention for hemangioma is indicated, what is the first-line treatment?

Corticosteroids (PO or IV)
(2–3 mg/kg/day)

Or

Propranolol (various routes)

(inappropriate in infants with high risk for cerebrovascular incidents)

Which hemangiomas require treatment?
(3)

1. Life or function threat
   (CHF, airway, vision)
2. Deformity issues (lip, nose, ear)
   & very large facial ones
3. Ulcerations

Why is Kasabach–Merritt syndrome important to know about?

Because this vascular tumor often causes a life-threatening consumptive coagulopathy

What is Kasabach–Merritt syndrome due to?

A rapidly growing congenital vascular tumor

(*NOT* a hemangioma, but it was previously thought to be one!)

Where on the body do the tumors that cause Kasabach–Merritt syndrome occur?

Superficial/skin

Or

Deep/visceral

(*just about anywhere*)

What is the "syndrome" part of Kasabach–Merritt syndrome? (3 components)

The vascular tumor

+

Thrombocytopenia due to platelet trapping

+

Consumptive coagulopathy

What is the prognosis for Kasabach–Merritt syndrome patients?

Not good –
High mortality

What kinds of tumors are responsible for Kasabach–Merritt syndrome? (2)

Tufted angioma

&

Kaposiform hemangioendothelioma

How is Kasabach–Merritt syndrome (or the vascular tumor that could cause it) treated?

Many techniques, depending on size & location:
1. Systemic corticosteroids
2. Alpha interferon & vincristine
3. Surgical excision/arterial embolization
4. Radiotherapy

When Kasabach–Merritt syndrome is recognized, how urgent is it to begin treatment?

Emergency!

Vascular malformations are not tumorous growths, but rather errors in the way a structure grew. Vascular malformations occur in what types of vessels?

All types
(arteries, veins, capillaries, lymphatics)

What is a "combined" vascular malformation?

Vein

+

one of the other vessel types is involved in the malformation

Which type of vascular malformation has the potential for serious blood loss?

Arteriovenous malformation (AVM)

(It is the only type with fast flow/ serious pressure)

What is the classic example of a capillary malformation?

Port-wine stain

(aka nevus flammeus)

What are the common names for a nevus simplex?

"Stork bite"
"Angel kiss"
"Salmon patch"

What is the usual course of a nevus simplex?

They fade in time

Port-wine stains are most common on what part of the body?

The face

What is the natural course of a port-wine stain?

• They get darker & thicker over time
• They "grow with the child" (continue to cover the same portions of the face as the child ages)

What is a port-wine stain?

Malformation in the upper dermis of "mature" capillaries

"Port-wine stains" have two other names in medicine. What are they?

Capillary malformation

&

Nevus flammeus
(this term is rarely used in current literature)

Do capillary malformations fade as the child ages?

No
(They usually worsen!)

Do capillary malformations develop & become visible weeks to months after birth?

No –
They are present at birth, although they may be light

How common is the capillary malformation in newborns?

Three per thousand

(3:1000)

How useful is laser treatment for port-wine stain?

Good
(The lesion is superficial – "pulsed dye" laser is used)

If there is a port-wine stain in either the V1 or V2 distribution, what ocular complication should you worry about?

Glaucoma

For those of you who don't remember . . .

V1 – forehead & around eye onto upper nose
V2 – cheek, upper lip, nasal ala

Capillary malformation is present in what part of the body?

The dermis

If a child has a port-wine stain (capillary malformation) in the V1 distribution, is it safe to assume that he or she has Sturge-Weber syndrome?

No! –
Only 5–10 % will have Sturge-Weber

What *is* Sturge-Weber syndrome?
  (3 categories of findings)

1. Cutaneous findings (port-wine stain, soft tissue & skeletal hypertrophy)
2. Ocular findings (glaucoma, vascular anomalies)
3. CNS findings (leptomeningeal malformations, cerebral atrophy, cortical calcification beneath malformation)

What consequences of the CNS problems of Sturge-Weber are commonly seen?

- **Hemiparesis**
- **Seizures (70 %)**
- **MR (50 %)**

(3)

A patient is diagnosed with Sturge-Weber syndrome. What will you see on the MRI of the brain?
(3)

- **Cerebral atrophy**
- **Enlarged choroid plexus**
- **Calcification in the cortex beneath the malformation (sometimes called "tram track" appearance)**

Which is more common – port-wine stain or Sturge-Weber syndrome?

Port-wine stain

(Remember, less than 10 % will have Sturge-Weber)

Port-wine stain (or capillary malformation) on an extremity may suggest that your patient has one of *which two* malformation syndromes?

Klippel-Trenaunay

Or

Parkes Weber syndromes

Which of the extremity port-wine stain syndromes is more concerning? Why?

- **Parkes Weber syndrome**
- **It involves a-v fistulas**

What complications are most likely with Parkes Weber syndrome?
(2)

CHF (high output)

&

Limb problems
(limb length disparity, ulcerations, progressive enlargement of limb)

Does the appearance of the port-wine stain on the extremity help you to anticipate how much the extremity will be affected in either Klippel or Parkes syndromes?

No –
Not at all

Klippel-Trenaunay syndrome usually affects what part of the body?

Lower extremity

The complications and associated findings of Klippel-Trenaunay syndrome involve what two general types of problems?

1. Hypertrophy of affected body areas
2. Venous stasis – DVT, recurrent cellulitis, pain, swelling

What proportion of hemangiomas are present at birth?

About 60 % –
The rest will present by 1–2 months

What is the *most common* complication of hemangiomas?

Ulceration

What are the three syndromes associated with hemangiomas?

1. **Diffuse neonatal hemangiomatosis (>4 hemangiomas)**
2. **LUMBAR/PELVIS syndrome (associated with lumbosacral hemangiomas)**
3. **PHACES**

   Posterior fossa malformations
   Hemangiomas
   Arterial anomalies (intracerebral)
   Cardiac anomalies/ coarctation
   Eye abnormalities
   Sternal defects

What problems are seen in the hemangioma syndrome associated with segmental perineal hemangiomas?

Lower body hemangioma/ cutaneous defects
Urogenital ulcers & anomalies
Myelopathy
Bony deformities
Anorectal & arterial anomalies
Renal anomalies

Perineal hemangioma
External genitalia malformations
Lipomyelomeningocele
Vesicorenal abnormalities
Imperforate anus
Skin tag

Is it possible for a vascular malformation to produce a consumptive coagulopathy?

Yes –
But it's very unusual! usually takes decades of growth to do this

Do café-au-lait spots sometimes develop into malignancies?

No!

Are café-au-lait spots associated with a risk of developing malignancies in other organs?

By themselves, no –

(If they are associated with neurofibromatosis, then some malignancies can develop)

How common are café-au-lait spots in the general population?

Common –
About 20 % have them

(Should have only one or two spots, though)

What qualifies as a "giant" congenital melanocytic nevus (CMN)?

>20 cm diameter

What types of cells are found in CMN?

Melanocytes

(makes sense!)

What is bad about having a giant CMN?

**10 % risk of melanoma –
50 % of the melanomas develop in the first 10 years of life!**

(+ Significant risk of neurocutaneous melanosis – nevi & leptomeningeal tumors often leading to melanoma)

How is a small CMN defined?

<1.5 cm diameter

If a CMN is between 1.5 & 20 cm in diameter, what do you call it?

Medium CMN

(makes sense again – amazing!)

What is the risk of developing melanoma in a small- or medium-sized CMN?

**Minimal –
And most develop after puberty**

Which large CMN lesions tell you that your patient may have a neural problem?

Those covering the midline of the back or scalp

What neural abnormalities are most likely with a giant midline CMN?

1. Spinal dysraphism
2. Dandy-Walker syndrome
   (or other posterior fossa issues)
3. Neurocutaneous melanosis

When can small- or medium-sized CMN also be associated with significant risk of neurocutaneous melanosis and melanoma?

When there are >3 of them

How do you diagnose neurocutaneous melanosis, if you suspect it?

Scan the head & spine

If your patient has *six or more* café-au-lait macules, what should you suspect?

Neurofibromatosis

What does a speckled lentiginous nevus look like?

Chocolate chip cookie – tan background with little dark spots

What is the significance of having a speckled lentiginous nevus (chocolate chip cookie lesion)?

Usually none –
There have been reports of melanoma developing in them, though

(sometimes electively removed for that reason)

What is the other name for a speckled lentiginous nevus (other than chocolate chip cookie lesion)?

Nevus spilus

How is nevus spilus usually managed?

Observation
(sometimes electively removed depending on size & location due to uncertain, very small, melanoma risk)

Is it worrisome if something that looks like a nevus spilus develops during childhood (wasn't present at birth)?

No –
They often do that

There are three types of nevi that develop in the epidermis. What are they?

1. Linear verrucous (means "warty")
2. Inflammatory linear verrucous
3. Nevus sebaceous

Are linear verrucous epidermal nevi warty?

Yes –
Just like the name says. They start out flat (either pink or dark) & then develop a warty surface

How is an inflammatory linear verrucous epidermal nevus (ILVEN) different from the regular kind?	Deeper red – Otherwise the same
Is it common for epidermal nevi to be pretty large or have multiple parts?	Yes – Sometimes they follow the skin lines
Nevus sebaceous is actually a hamartoma in the epidermal skin. What is the hamartoma made of? (What tissue types?)	Sebaceous & Apocrine glands
Where do nevus sebaceous usually occur?	Scalp or face
If a nevus sebaceous occurs on the scalp, will the hair grow through it?	No
What does a nevus sebaceous look like?	• **Waxy plaque (on scalp or face)** • **Various shapes** • **Pink, yellow, or orange**
What is the usual course for a nevus sebaceous? (2 aspects)	• It becomes warty at puberty (!) & sometimes enlarges • 10 % risk of basal cell carcinoma over lifetime Mnemonic: Basal cell has a pearly appearance & so does nevus sebaceous
What is the recommended management of nevus sebaceous?	Elective excision before puberty (risk for basal cell begins at puberty)
The darkly pigmented nevi are associated with the risk of which malignancy?	Melanoma (unless there are just one or two small-medium CMNs)
Which type of nevus is associated with basal cell carcinoma?	Nevus sebaceous ("of Jadassohn" is technically part of the name for these)
Are linear verrucous nevi associated with the risk for later malignancy?	No

What is the most common type
of diaper dermatitis?

Irritant!

What age infant is most likely
to develop diaper dermatitis?

9–12 months

What are the three factors that conspire
to cause diaper dermatitis,
of various sorts?

1. Physical (friction damage to very
   well-hydrated skin)
2. Chemical – urine & feces combine
   to activate fecal enzymes that
   damage the skin
3. Microbial – candida & other
   microbes like the warm, moist
   diaper environment

Who has more diaper rash – breast-fed
or bottle-fed babies?

Bottle fed –
Has to do with higher stool pH

Since fecal enzymes do a lot of the skin
damage in diaper dermatitis, what do
you think the relationship is between
stool frequency and the development
of diaper dermatitis?

↑ stooling
↑ diaper dermatitis

**What is the hallmark of irritant
diaper dermatitis?**

**Skin folds are spared
(that skin was protected from
contact)**

Can papules & erosions be part
of irritant diaper dermatitis?

Yes

**What is the mainstay of treatment
for irritant-based diaper dermatitis?**

**Barrier ointments containing zinc
oxide**

How is the presentation of candidal
diaper dermatitis different
from irritant based?

- Deeper red
- Likes skin folds
  (but may not be in them in all
  cases)
- Forms satellite lesions *outside*
  the diaper area

If a child has recently been treated
with an antibiotic, which type of diaper
rash is most likely?

Candidal

Which familial disorder creates an itchy rash in the diaper area and other places with skin folds?	Seborrheic dermatitis
If the diaper area looks like it's developing hypopigmentation – like vitiligo – what is it more likely to be?	Post-inflammatory hypopigmentation due to seborrheic dermatitis
A very-well-defined red rash in the diaper area, often with a shiny somewhat thickened plaque appearance, is likely to be _____?	Psoriasis
If a child develops psoriatic diaper dermatitis, is it safe to assume he or she will develop regular psoriasis later?	No – Often don't
A peeling, desquamating red rash in the diaper area, in a child running a fever, can be a tipoff to which disorder?	Kawasaki's (The diaper area often peels before the extremities do)
A diaper rash common in older babies develops from moisture and occlusion, and sometimes bacterial infections. What is it called? (multiple erythematous papules/pustules)	Folliculitis
If an older baby is having recurrent episodes of folliculitis in the diaper area, what is the likely etiology?	Perianal staph or strep colonization
A bottom that looks like it's covered in "flaking paint," like a building in poor repair, is characteristic of what nutrition-related problem?	Kwashiorkor (the mainly *protein*-deficient form of malnutrition)
Which is more common as a cause of skin lesions – dietary zinc deficiency or the genetic condition that impairs zinc absorption?	Dietary deficiency
Zinc deficiency causes what characteristic skin problems in infants?	Perioral & perianal rash

What is the name of the genetic condition that impairs zinc absorption, causing skin lesions?	Acrodermatitis enteropathica Mnemonic: enteropathica = gut pathology acrodermatitis = skin inflammation at the ends of the body!
A diaper rash that looks like seborrheic diaper dermatitis (in folds), but which also has *petechiae* could be what very important to diagnose disorder?	**Langerhans cell histiocytosis**
Why is it important to diagnose Langerhans cell histiocytosis?	Because rapid treatment of multi-system disease has a *much* better prognosis (multi-system disease is malignant)
How is the diagnosis of Langerhans cell histiocytosis made?	Biopsy
What are the main features of atopic dermatitis, meaning what do you see clinically?	Xerosis (dryness) & Pruritis (itchiness)
What percentage of pediatric patients will be affected by atopic dermatitis?	>10 %
What percentage of people with atopic dermatitis has symptoms within the first year of life?	60 %
If atopic dermatitis presents for the first time in someone aged 10, what should you consider?	**Another diagnosis – It is very rare for it to present so late**
During acute exacerbations of atopic dermatitis, what do you expect to see in terms of skin lesions?	Redness, weeping, crusting, & scaling +/− vesicles (also excoriation, due to the patient scratching)
What chronic changes often occur with atopic dermatitis over time?	Lichenification & Changes in pigmentation

What is lichenification of the skin?	Skin thickening and increased skin markings (little lines in the skin)
Atopic dermatitis has three phases that differ in terms of the skin usually affected. What are the three phases?	Infantile (to 18 months) Childhood (18 months – puberty) Adolescent & adult phase
In infantile atopic dermatitis, where does the rash usually begin?	Cheeks or scalp
What part of the extremities is mainly affected in infantile atopic dermatitis?	<u>Extensor</u> surfaces (different from the usual pattern)
Which part of the infant's skin is conspicuously spared in infantile atopic dermatitis?	The diaper area (probably due to moisture)
Where is atopic dermatitis usually found in the childhood phase?	<u>Flexural</u> surfaces – Including neck
When is lichenification first seen in atopic dermatitis? (during which phase)	Childhood
A weepy, excoriated, erythematous skin area bilaterally in the popliteal fossa suggests what disorder?	Childhood atopic dermatitis
What are the hallmarks of the adolescent/ adult phase for atopic dermatitis?	Flexor area problems (continued) & Hand, foot, & periocular involvement
What are the three mainstays of treatment for atopic dermatitis exacerbations?	1. Moisturizer/emollients 2. Avoid irritants (triggers) 3. Treat active inflammation with steroids or immunomodulators (topically)
Which medications are first-line therapy for atopic dermatitis exacerbations?	Steroids

Which two parts of the body should virtually *always* be treated with low-potency steroids, when steroids are used?	Face & Diaper area (because the occlusion increases absorption/potency significantly)
Patients with atopic dermatitis are at significantly increased risk for what types of skin infections? (2 general categories)	• Secondary bacterial infections • Viral disseminated skin infections
What are some typical irritant triggers for atopic dermatitis flares?	Wool, dyes, fragrances
When should topical immunomodulators be used in atopic dermatitis? (2 conditions)	• Steroids & other more conservative things failed • Child is older than 2 years
Do topical immunomodulators work best for flares, or for maintenance management?	Maintenance
Which two immunosuppressants, available in topical preparations, are sometimes used for atopic dermatitis?	Pimecrolimus & Tacrolimus (Pimecrolimus is preferred due to less systemic absorption)
Do antihistamines have a role in atopic dermatitis regimens?	Yes – Mainly at bedtime to facilitate sleep (To decrease itching that can interfere with sleep)
Atopic dermatitis is usually considered to be a nuisance condition. What significant health/developmental effects can it have?	*Altered sleep patterns* Decreased/slowed growth Psychosocial impact
An atopic dermatitis patient presents with fever, irritability, and diffuse erosions of the skin – worst in his typical spots for dermatitis. What is the likely diagnosis?	Eczema herpeticum

What is eczema herpeticum?

Diffuse HSV eruption that can develop in patients with atopic dermatitis

How should you treat eczema herpeticum?

Usually IV acyclovir
(very mild cases may only require oral)

If the diffuse lesions of eczema herpeticum are on the face, what must you consider?

Ophthalmological involvement (get an ophtho consult!)

What is the most common significant contact allergen?

Metal (usually nickel)

What are some other common contact irritants that we often put on our skin?
(2 groups)

- Topical medicine & its preservatives
- Fragrances & dyes

Which contact irritant is usually encountered unintentionally, in the outdoor environment?

Plant resins

(e.g., urushiol – poison ivy's irritant)

The keys to diagnosing contact dermatitis are what characteristics of the rash?
(2)

1. Itchy
2. Odd shapes/patterns

What is the "id" reaction?

Generalized papular dermatitis

Or

Periumbilical dermatitis

(usually a reaction to nickel)

How early in life would you expect to see contact dermatitis?

6 months or older

Should you treat contact dermatitis with systemic steroids?

Only if it's severe, very large area, or near the eyes

If you are treating contact dermatitis with systemic steroids, how long should the treatment course be?

About 3 weeks –
It takes that long for the reaction to settle down

| How are typical contact dermatitis cases handled? | Topical steroids
Moisturizers
Antihistamines |

| What is keratosis pilaris? | Basically, rough skin due to follicles forming little papules

(The skin protein called "keratin" forms hard plugs within hair follicles) |

| On what part of the body is keratosis pilaris usually seen? | Extensor surfaces
Buttocks
Cheeks (of the face!) |

| Which patients are most likely to develop keratosis pilaris? | Atopic dermatitis patients
&
Those with dry skin |

| If a patient would like treatment for keratosis pilaris, what can be done? | Keratolytic agents may help

(lactic acid cream or topical retinoids) |

| What is ichthyosis vulgaris? | Scaly skin
(literally fish-like skin)
With increased lines on palms & soles |

| How does a person develop ichthyosis vulgaris? | Inherited –
Autosomal dominant |

| At what age are the skin changes of ichthyosis vulgaris usually noticeable? | First year of life |

| If you have an ichthyosis vulgaris patient who would like to move to a better climate to improve the condition, should you recommend Santa Fe (cool & dry) or the Gulf Coast (warm & humid)? | Gulf Coast –
It improves with warmth & humidity |

| Ichthyosis vulgaris often co-occurs with what other skin condition? | 50 % have atopic dermatitis |

A patient presents with platelike scale on the shins, and the plates are dark. What skin disorders might that be?

Ichthyosis vulgaris

(plate color varies – usually dark)

How is pityriasis alba different from vitiligo?

It is less well defined, and it is hypopigmented rather than depigmented

(total loss of pigment in vitiligo)

What does pityriasis alba look like?

Vague hypopigmented macules – Usually on the face

(It is especially noticeable in times of sun exposure, because the skin won't tan as well as the surrounding skin)

Which patients most often develop pityriasis alba?

Dry skin

   Or

Atopic dermatitis patients

What is the natural course of pityriasis alba?

Goes away in time (can be several years)

How is pityriasis alba different from pityriasis rosea?
   (4 ways)

- Alba is light (not red or darker than usual)
- Alba does not follow a viral illness
- Alba occurs mainly on the face (not trunk)
- No "herald patch" or Christmas tree rash pattern

How is pityriasis alba treated?

Just moisturize & sunscreen (to prevent suntan around the lesion making it more obvious)

Some patients complain of red and itchy spots, at the onset of a pityriasis alba lesion. Is there a satisfactory treatment for these?

Mild topical corticosteroid

What are some common areas for the depigmentation of vitiligo?	Perioral Dorsal hands Knees Genitals
Vitiligo is sometimes associated with autoimmune diseases. Which autoimmune disease most often co-occurs with vitiligo?	Autoimmune thyroid dysfunction
Will the skin changes of vitiligo go away in time?	Sometimes – But repigmentation often occurs in a "freckled" or "follicular" pattern (Cycles of depigmentation, followed by stable periods, occur in some patients. The process often stops entirely after a time, for reasons that are not known)
What is the significance of "halo nevi?"	Associated with later development of vitiligo
What does a halo nevus look like?	Dark nevus with a light hypopigmented area surrounding it
How is vitiligo treated? (3)	Topical steroids Immunomodulators Phototherapy (none are very effective)
If a patient presents with vitiligo, what should you most want to investigate?	Review of systems & family history for autoimmune diseases
How common is vitiligo?	**1 % of population!**
Large, silvery plaques, with tiny pinpoints of bleeding if you disturb them, means a patient has what disorder?	**Psoriasis**
Sometimes psoriasis lesions will spread into unusual areas, following trauma to the area. What is this phenomenon called?	Koebner phenomenon

Typical changes in the nails that go with psoriasis are . . . ? (2)	1. Pitting 2. Onycholysis (separation from the nail bed) *Popular photo item*
Where do psoriatic plaques usually form?	Areas of high friction – Knees, elbows, sacrum, & scalp, umbilicus Mnemonic: Imagine someone who always wears a hat to make the friction idea work with the scalp!
Can psoriasis be found in intertriginous areas?	Ordinarily, no – But in "inverse psoriasis" it is!
How is psoriasis treated with topical preparations?	Steroids Immunomodulators Tar preparations
Which topical vitamin prep is often helpful in managing psoriasis?	Topical vitamin D (e.g., calcipotriene or Dovonex®)
What usually determines whether systemic therapy for psoriasis is warranted?	% of body affected – Large % (>20 %) or functional impairment means systemic therapy (along with degree of joint involvement – psoriatic arthritis)
Which systemic treatments are commonly used in psoriasis treatment? (3)	• UV (with or without psoralen as a primer) • Methotrexate • Cyclosporine
What is guttate psoriasis?	**Temporary psoriasis that breaks out in response to a strep infection**
Does strep pharyngitis precipitate guttate psoriasis?	Yes – Any strep infection can cause it
How is guttate psoriasis treated?	**Treat the strep & it will usually go away**

How do you recognize guttate psoriasis?

"Drop-like" papules and plaques of erythema all over the patient – especially on the trunk – with a little scale on the papules/plaques

("guttate" means drop-like)

Is guttate psoriasis more common in kids or adults?

Kids

(May recur with subsequent strep infections)

Guttate psoriasis looks a lot like secondary syphilis. How could you try to differentiate them?

Less palm & sole involvement in guttate psoriasis

Where does seborrheic dermatitis develop *on infants*?

Scalp

&

Intertriginous areas

What is the commonly used name for infantile seborrheic dermatitis?

Cradle cap

How is infantile seborrheic dermatitis treated?

Mineral oil/emollients

&

Antifungals (topically) & topical hydrocortisone, as needed

What is the natural course of infantile seborrheic dermatitis?

Resolves in less than a year (usually by 6 months)

What age groups does seborrhea affect?

Infants
Adolescents
Adults

(skips school aged!!!)

If a school-aged child presents with dandruff, what is the likely disorder?

Tinea capitis –
Seborrhea doesn't really affect school-aged kids!

What is the mainstay of treatment for seborrheic dandruff?	OTC shampoos – Must rotate type every 2 weeks for them to be effective
	(Options: tar, salicylic acid, zinc, selenium, ketoconazole)
For seborrhea affecting the face, what medications or treatments will help? (3)	Moisturizers Low-potency topical steroids Topical antifungals
What percentage of adolescents has some acne vulgaris?	85 %

What percentage of adolescents will have some scarring due to acne by age 18?

25 %
(more than you would think!)

Which bacterium is involved in the formation of acne vulgaris lesions?	Propionibacterium acnes
How does an acne lesion get started?	Abnormal shedding of the lining in the hair follicle blocks the "pilosebaceous unit"
Which hormone is most directly involved in the genesis of acne?	DHEAS – (dehydroepiandrosterone sulfate)
	It stimulates gland development & sebum production
What kind of a bacterium is propionibacterium?	Anaerobic gram + diphtheroid
	(Remember that eria is also a diphtheroid!)
How does the inflammatory part of the acne process mainly begin?	Neutrophils attacking *P. acnes* damage the follicle wall, releasing content into the surrounding tissue
What are the noninflammatory types of acne lesions?	Open
	&
	Closed Comedones (black & white heads)

What is the main determinant
of aggressiveness in treatment approach
for acne?

Scarring

&

Potential for scarring

At what age does adolescent-type
acne begin?

8–9 years old

(That's when DHEAS secretion
increases)

Which type of acne lesion is likely
to produce scarring?

Acneiform cyst

(a painful, deep dermal pus nodule)

On what part of the face or body does
acne usually begin?

Central face
(usually with open & closed
comedones)

If acne develops in a young child,
between age 1 and 7 years, what should
you do?

Endocrine work-up

Why would a bone age be helpful in
evaluating early-onset acne?

Androgens affect the bone age –
it is an indirect measure of androgens

When should oral antibiotics be used
for acne?

Moderate-to-severe *inflammatory*
acne

(If moderate, it needs to fail topicals
first)

How is moderate acne defined?
(This is the most important category to
remember, of all of the acne categories)

20–100 comedones

Or

15–50 inflammatory lesions

Or

30–125 total lesions

**(Just remember that less than
these numbers = mild, more than
these numbers = severe)**

**How many cysts are enough to qualify
a patient as having "severe acne?"**

Six or more

How many comedones would qualify a patient as having severe acne?	**>100**
When are topical antibiotics indicated for acne?	**Mild-to-moderate** *inflammatory* **acne**
When would benzoyl peroxide be an appropriate acne treatment?	**Mild-moderate inflammatory acne**
Most topical acne medications have what possible annoying side effects?	**Irritation/redness** + **Drying & peeling**
Which acne treatment is recommended for both inflammatory *and* *noninflammatory* **acne?**	**Topical retinoids**
Why are topical retinoids helpful for acne?	**Normalizes the shedding of the follicular epithelium,** *preventing comedones* **(& fixing existing comedones!)**
How are synthetic retinoids different from "all-trans retinoic acid?"	Improved efficacy & *Decreased side effects!*
Which antibiotics are most commonly used for acne? (common topical & oral agents are the same)	**Erythromycin** & **Cyclines (tetracycline, doxycycline, minocycline)**
Although antibiotics kill propionibacterium acne, much of their effect is due to what other action (shared by most acne meds)?	Reduced inflammation
A patient presents to your office for acne. She is 14 years old, and has ten scattered erythematous papules or pustules on her forehead & cheeks. She has comedones on her nose, numbering about 15. How should you treat her?	**Mild acne –** **Topical retinoid** *Benzoyl peroxide* **Topical antibiotic (some combination of these)**

A 17-year-old male presents to you for control of his acne. He has seven cystic lesions, scattered pustules, and numerous comedones. What treatments are indicated for him?

(3)

- Oral antibiotic
- Topical retinoid & antibiotic
- Derm referral for possible oral isotretinoin

For mild acne on the boards, the first-line treatment is usually considered to be _____?

Benzoyl peroxide!

If an oral antibiotic is indicated for acne, should you use a topical antibiotic as well?

Yes

What is the most common annoying side effect of tetracycline medications?

Sun sensitivity

When is it appropriate to send an acne patient to the dermatologist?

Moderate acne not responding to initial meds

Or

Severe acne

Should pediatricians give systemic retinoids?

Generally not –
Leave that for derm

Why is systemic retinoid treatment so good for treating acne?

It treats _all_ of the things that contribute to acne

(inflammation, bacteria, sebum production, & follicular keratinization)

Use of systemic retinoids has been linked to what psychiatric issue?

Depression

Do systemic retinoids still cause cutaneous side effects?

**Yes –
Erythema
Dry skin, lips, eyes
Photosensitivity
Epistaxis (due to dry mucous membranes)**

What effect do systemic retinoids sometimes have on the hair?	**Hair loss/thinning**
What visual side effect sometimes accompanies systemic retinoid use?	**Poor night vision (and you thought vitamin A was supposed to help your eyes!)**
	(Isotretinoin replaces retinoic acid on rod cell receptors of the retina, responsible for low light vision – that is why this effect sometimes occurs – and is a good way to remember the side effect!)
Systemic retinoids are associated with what CNS neurological effect (just like hypervitaminosis A is)?	**Headache/pseudotumor cerebri**
What musculoskeletal effects go with systemic retinoid therapy? (3)	1. **Myalgia** 2. **Calcification of tendons/ ligaments** 3. **Hyperostosis**
Although short-term use of systemic retinoids in kids shouldn't make this side effect a big deal, what alteration of the lipid profile should you be aware of?	**Hypertriglyceridemia**
Monitoring of which organ is usually routinely conducted for patients taking systemic retinoids?	**Liver**
Vitamin A products are well known for their teratogenicity. What are the rules about contraception & pregnancy testing for patients taking/considering isotretinoin? (4)	1. **Two negative pregnancy tests before starting** 2. **Two effective forms of birth control** 3. **Double birth control for 1 month before & after therapy** 4. **Monthly pregnancy tests for refills**
Why are oral contraceptives helpful in the treatment of acne?	They decrease androgens

Which patients are candidates for oral contraceptive acne treatment?
(4)

1. Failed standard treatment
2. Acne related to menses
3. OCs desired for gyn reasons anyway
4. Inflammatory acne on lower face & neck area

A patient suddenly develops sheets of pustules on the trunk – all are in the same stage of development. What is the likely disorder?

Acneiform eruption
(usually due to a medication)

Which meds are most likely to cause an acneiform eruption?
(4 groups)

Steroids
Seizure meds
Lithium
TB meds (isoniazid & rifampin)

If oral contraceptives improve acne by decreasing androgens, will androgen-blocking medications also work?

Yes –
For example spironolactone is sometimes used this way

Where would the dermatophytes that cause tinea corporis prefer to live? Florida or Arizona?

Florida –
They enjoy the heat & humidity

Mnemonic:
Think of some dermatophytes in lounge chairs by a condo in Boca Raton!

All of the fungi that cause dermatophyte infections have phyton in the name, except which one?

Microsporum canis

If a ringworm lesion has papules or pustules at the edge, is it probably secondarily infected?

No –
They're usually just inflammatory

Why might a ringworm lesion look like a target?

The edge enlarges while the center clears
(scaling edge, round shape)

To definitively diagnose tinea corporis, what will you need to do?

Fungal culture or KOH prep of the "leading edge"

(Leading edge = edge of the lesion)

Combinations of steroids & antifungals have been popular for treating dermatophyte infections. What is the current treatment recommendation?

Topical antifungal BID for a month

(Combos were expensive & had an increased risk of complications & recurrence)

What must you be sure to tell the person applying medication to a tinea corporis site?
   (2 items)

1. It can be spread by skin-to-skin contact (!) – wear a glove
2. Apply to the surrounding area (1 cm around the lesion) to eliminate the infection

When would systemic treatment of ringworm lesions be advisable?

Immunocompromised

   Or

Large area involved with poor response to topicals

What is nummular dermatitis – also known as nummular eczema?

Roundish lesions of eczema that occur on the extremities

What should you consider before treating a case of nummular dermatitis?

Whether fungal or bacterial infection is present

(culture &/or KOH prep)

Is the treatment for nummular dermatitis/eczema different from the treatment for regular eczema?

No

What is the common name for urticaria?

Hives

What causes urticaria?

Histamine release from mast cells (in response to antigen triggers)

A "transient" or "acute" outbreak of hives should last how long?

<6 weeks

(6 weeks! Sounds like a long time to have hives!)

What is it called if a patient develops hives intermittently for more than 6 weeks?

Chronic idiopathic urticaria

What are typical triggers for acute urticaria?
   (3 categories)

1. New meds or food
2. Infections
3. Stings/bites

If a patient has hives, then they resolve, but a dusky, bruised-looking area remains, what does that mean?

Usually nothing –
Leaky capillaries in a hive often leak some blood cells producing bruising

Will the redness that goes with a hive blanch?

Yes

What is an important clue to diagnosing hives, in terms of their duration & location?

• Most common on upper chest/face/upper arms
• Last <24 h in one place

Why might urticaria be confused with the lesions of erythema multiforme?

The lesions may be various sizes, & sometimes have central clearing or dusky centers

(but they are itchy and short-lived, unlike EM)

What odd mechanism sometimes causes hives?

Mechanical/physical phenomena (usually pressure or cold)

How are hives treated?
   (3 components)

• H_1 & H_2 blockers
• Oral steroids only if airway issue/more severe reaction
• Remove trigger, if possible

What physical stimulus sometimes causes acne?

Pressure

How long do the lesions of erythema multiforme last?

Several days
(in one spot, that is)

To qualify as erythema multiforme *minor*, lesions must be limited to skin and _____?

One mucous membrane surface

What is the most common trigger for erythema multiforme minor?

Recurrent herpes simplex infection/outbreak

(frequently tested!)

(Mycoplasma infection is another common association!)

What should the center of an erythema multiforme minor (EMM) lesion look like?

Dusky

Classically, what does an EMM lesion look like?

Target-like with three zones of color change –
pale, red, & dusky

Dusky means a little dark, usually a dark red or blue-violet color

The pale ring sits between the dusky center & the red rim at the outside

What aspects of EMM's appearance can help you to make the diagnosis?
(3 aspects)

- Symmetric
- Most commonly found on distal body parts
- At most, one mucous membrane affected

A patient with a history of recurrent, painful, vesicular eruptions presents with a "funny rash" on the hands & legs – red & pale. What is the likely diagnosis?

Erythema multiforme minor

(80 % of cases are related to HSV)

Skin-colored to violaceous nodules appear on a patient's shins. They are tender to touch. What is the likely diagnosis?

Erythema nodosum

Skin-colored to violaceous nodules appear on the dorsum of a patient's hands & feet. They are not tender. They are not scaly. What are they?

Granuloma annulare

(Tinea corporis looks similar, but has scale)

Why are the lesions of granuloma annulare raised, and why can't they have scale?

The process is in the dermis

Which patient group is most likely to get granuloma annulare?

Girls

(Children & females are most often affected)

Does granuloma annulare have a risk of malignancy?

No

How is granuloma annulare treated?	"Tincture" of time – Just wait a while and it will go away (takes months to years, though)
Is granuloma annulare caused by immune cell dysfunction?	No – It's not a true granuloma (the cause is not clear)
If a patient has numerous granuloma annulare lesions, what should you consider?	**Diabetes**

After the main rash of pityriasis rosea has broken out, what does it look a lot like?
    (2 for your differential)
	Guttate psoriasis
	
	    Or
	
	Secondary syphilis

Which types of dermatophyte infections will fluoresce with a Wood's lamp?	Ones that come from pets (Microsporum canis)
What percentage of dermatophyte infections are the fluorescing type?	**Only 10 %**
Which ethnic group is most often affected by tinea capitis?	African-Americans (kids around age 5 most often affected)
What tip-offs will you see in the hair of tinea capitis patients?	**Broken hairs** **Or** **Black dots & alopecia (the black dots are hairs that are *very short*)**
Some patients develop a big boggy area around a tinea capitis infection. What is this?	**A "kerion"** **(an inflammatory mass that goes away when the infection is over)**
An itchy red scaly area in the shape of a coin on the head is probably what diagnosis?	**Tinea capitis**
Are pustules a feature of tinea capitis infection?	Sometimes – Or they could indicate superinfection

On physical exam, what important associated finding goes with tinea capitis?

Occipital or post-auricular lymphadenopathy

What does the term "alopecia" refer to?

Hair loss –
Regardless of the cause

What is the most common cause of alopecia in children?

Tinea capitis

What is the main concern if a kerion has formed?

Possible scarring

Effective treatment of tinea capitis requires?
(2)

1. Systemic antifungals (it's in the follicle, so topical alone won't work)
2. Antifungal shampoo – for family members, too

In addition to treatment, what else must you do to successfully treat a patient with tinea capitis?

Examine & treat classmates and playmates if <8 years old

Which systemic antifungal should you use to treat tinea capitis?

They all have equal efficacy – doesn't matter

What is alopecia areata?

Non-scarring alopecia that runs in families

After an episode of alopecia areata, will the hair grow back?

Often yes,
but recurrences are common

What important group of disorders is associated with alopecia areata?

Autoimmune disease
(thyroid, vitiligo, etc.)

Is alopecia areata common in kids?

1 %
(pretty common)

Is there any obvious inflammation involved in alopecia areata?

No –
The areas are asymptomatic except for hair loss

If an area of hair loss is also red or scaly, does this rule-out alopecia areata?

Yes –
Should be "smooth as a baby's bottom"

Is alopecia areata treatable?	Somewhat – Immunosuppressives are helpful (topicals or intralesionals)
How is alopecia areata totalis different from regular alopecia?	• All hair on the head is lost • Hair regrowth is unlikely
What nail finding is nearly always present in alopecia areata patients?	Pitting or thinning
What is traction alopecia?	Partial or complete hair loss in areas of traction (tight braids are usually responsible)
Will areas damaged by traction alopecia regrow?	Usually – If the traction/trauma stops
What is telogen effluvium?	When significant amounts of hair are lost because the hair growth cycle synchronizes (so it all falls out at the same time!)
What causes hair growth to be unusually synchronized, making telogen effluvium possible?	Significant illness, surgery, physical stress, pregnancy (Note: The hair falls out 2–6 months later)
Does complete alopecia occur with telogen effluvium?	Generally, no
How is telogen effluvium treated?	Wait for it to grow again!
Does complete alopecia occur with telogen effluvium?	Not usually
How do you identify alopecia due to trichotillomania? (3)	• Unusual shape to the area • Well defined • Hair of multiple lengths
How is trichotillomania defined?	"Compulsive" pulling, twisting, or breaking of your own hair

Is trichotillomania limited to hair on the head?

Not necessarily –
Sometimes eyebrows & eyelashes are also involved

How is childhood trichotillomania treated?

- Behavioral modification
- Antidepressants

(prognosis for cure is better in kids than it is in adults)

The earliest signs of neurofibromatosis 1 occur in which body system? What are they?

- **Skin**
- **>5 café-au-lait spots & intertriginous freckling (axillary & inguinal)**

The axillary & inguinal freckling that is often seen in neurofibromatosis type 1 is also known by what eponymic name?

Crowe's sign

At what age are skin findings usually present for neurofibromatosis 1 patients?

Often present at birth, but definitely present before age 5

When do neurofibromas usually start to appear for neurofibroma patients?

Late childhood/
Early adolescence

Which type of neurofibroma is nearly always present at birth, for patients that have them, even if it's not obvious on physical exam?

"Plexiform"

(Pigmented, often hairy, and progressively enlarges)

Plexiform neurofibromas look a lot like _____?

CMN

Why is an ocular exam recommended if neurofibromatosis is suspected?

2 reasons –
1. Diagnosis – finding Lisch nodules is helpful
2. Optic gliomas are common & often asymptomatic

What are Lisch nodules? I just can't seem to remember!

Hamartomas in the iris

(can be clear, yellow, or brown, but on exams they are usually colored for easy identification)

What percentage of patients with neurofibromatosis will develop optic gliomas?	15 %

Although this is the dermatology section, which skeletal findings should you know are common for NF1?	Macrocephaly & Cervical-thoracic kyphosis/scoliosis

Which two skeletal findings are pathognomonic of NF1, although they don't occur in many patients?	**Sphenoid wing dysplasia** **&** **Pseudoarthrosis of tibia**

Some people have dark-colored nevi on their irises. How can you tell an iris nevus from a Lisch nodule?	**Lisch nodules are raised**

How common is it for neurofibromatosis patients to have Lisch nodules?	*Very* common – At least 50 % have them by age 6 years & nearly 100 % have them after puberty

Which CNS tumors are NF patients at increased risk to develop?	• *Acoustic schwannomas* • *Optic gliomas* (& other astrocytomas) • Meningiomas • Ependymomas

Do NF1 & NF2 come from the same genetic defect?	No – But both are due to loss of a tumor-suppressor gene (NF2 is chromosome 22) (NF1 is 17q11)

Which gene product is altered in NF2?	Schwannomin, which is also known as "Merlin" Mnemonic: Think of Merlin the magician changing into a "schwann" with a lot of lumps on it – from neurofibromas

Which protein is affected in NF1?	Neurofibromin
In addition to neurofibromatosis, which other genetic disorder causes café-au-lait spots?	**McCune-Albright syndrome**
What are the four main features of McCune-Albright syndrome?	1. *Café-au-lait macules* 2. *Precocious puberty* 3. Hyperthyroidism 4. Polyostotic fibrous dysplasia (misshapen bones)
Tuberous sclerosis is an autosomal dominant disorder when it is inherited. Is it usually inherited or sporadic?	**Sporadic** **(About 75 %)**
The most recognizable dermatological lesions of tuberous sclerosis, which are also present on the vast majority of patients (85 %), are what two lesions?	• Ash leaf spots (light-colored macules) • Facial angiofibromas (skin-colored to pink or yellow papules on the face)
What is a "Shagreen patch?"	A "connective tissue nevus" made of surplus collagen in the skin – *occurs in the lumbosacral area*
In addition to the lumbosacral area, where else are collagenomas or connective tissue nevi sometimes found?	On the forehead! (Called a "fibrous forehead plaque")
What is the other name for the facial angiofibromas that usually develop with tuberous sclerosis?	Adenoma sebaceum (This name is more commonly used, but less correct. It is neither an adenoma nor does it involve the sebaceous glands!)
Where does the adenoma sebaceum of tuberous sclerosis usually develop?	The face – Mainly nose, cheeks, and especially along the alar crease
What are the most common cutaneous manifestations of tuberous sclerosis? (4)	1. Hypopigmented macules 2. Facial angiofibromas 3. Fibromas (gums & near nails) 4. Collagenomas (lumbosacral & forehead)

In a photo, it could be difficult to differentiate adenoma sebaceum of tuberous sclerosis from acne. What is one helpful clue?

Adenoma sebaceum does *not* affect the forehead –
acne nearly always does

What percentage of tuberous sclerosis patients has intracerebral calcifications & mental retardation?

60 % have calcifications
60 % have intellectual disability

(Most patients with intellectual disability also have seizures)

Neurofibromatosis patients develop hamartomas of the iris. Where do tuberous sclerosis patients typically develop hamartomas?

The retina

(about 60 % get these)

Alteration of which two proteins (from which two chromosomes) results in tuberous sclerosis?

Hamartin (Chr 9)

&

Tuberin (Chr 16)

Incontinentia pigmenti is an uncommon disorder that affects several body systems, including the skin. What is important to know about the skin effects?

There are four phases:
1. Vesicles
2. Verrucous (warty)
3. Hyperpigmentation
4. Loss of pigment/atrophy

What other effects, in addition to skin findings, go with incontinentia pigmenti?

Ocular
Dental
CNS

(all neuroectodermal tissues)

When are the skin findings of incontinentia pigmenti usually evident?

The vesicular phase is noticeable at birth or within a few weeks

What is important to know about how you get incontinentia pigmenti?

It is *X-linked dominant*

(more females affected because it is often lethal in males!)

After the vesicular & verrucous phases are done (for incontinentia pigmenti), where will the skin be hyperpigmented?

Wherever the verrucous areas were –
Sometimes follows the skin lines, but doesn't have to

How long does the hyperpigmentation of incontinentia pigmenti last?

Usually until adolescence, then they fade (but may hypopigment or atrophy)

How is hypomelanosis of Ito different in appearance from incontinentia pigmenti?

- Affected areas are light from the beginning
- No multiple phases

Do hypomelanosis of Ito patients also have problems in other body systems, like incontinentia pigmenti?

Yes –
CNS, ocular, & skeletal (about 40 % of Ito patients have problems in these systems)

Erythema nodosum is classically seen on the shins. Where else is it often seen?

Back of the calves

&

On the thighs

What is erythema nodosum, in terms of its pathophysiology?

Panniculitis

(Inflammation in the subQ fat)

What is the most common precipitant of erythema nodosum in children?

Infections

What rheumatologic/connective tissue disorders are associated with erythema nodosum?

Sarcoid

&

IBD

When medications precipitate erythema nodosum, which medications are most likely to be at fault?

Sulfa

Or

Oral contraceptives

A genetic disorder that prevents proper zinc absorption leads to what dermatologic disorder?

Acrodermatitis enteropathica

When erythema nodosum is resolving, what will it look like?

Either –
1. The overall color lightens, or
2. The middle lightens first (same in erythema multiforme minor)

An infant is shown in a photo with a rash in the diaper area. It looks like "peeling paint." What cause of the diaper dermatitis does this suggest?

Protein malnutrition
(aka kwashiorkor)

Cystic fibrosis is always a popular pediatric topic – what is the main dermatological issue in CF?

Diffuse dermatitis

(Aquagenic skin wrinkling, in which papules form on the palms of CF patients in response to water exposure, then resolve over several hours, is a more rare, but an interesting phenomenon. The palms look a lot like hands usually do, if they've been submerged in water for a long time)

When are the skin findings of CF most likely to be seen?

Young infancy –
Because they are due to nutritional deficiencies caused by CF, which are then treated

Which nutritional issues are the main causes of CF-related dermatitis?

Zinc

&

Free fatty acids

(these deficiencies have usually been corrected in older children, so dermatitis is not seen in older age groups)

A very young infant is shown with an all-over erythematous dermatitis, and you correctly diagnose CF-related dermatitis. How quickly will the skin normalize if appropriate nutritional support is given?

Within days!

If a patient is diagnosed as having discoid lupus erythematosus, what should you tell him or her about the prognosis?

Initially, can't say –
Some have only skin findings, while others have systemic lupus

What does discoid lupus erythematosus look like?

- **Erythematous round lesions**
- **Often have central clearing**
- **Usually on face**

How can you clinically identify leukocytoclastic vasculitis in children? (This is a general category of vasculitis)	**Palpable purpura**
If the patient has been diagnosed with leukocytoclastic vasculitis, does that provide you with sufficient information about the etiology?	No – A whole range of things can trigger leukocytoclastic vasculitis
What is the most common cause of leukocytoclastic vasculitis in children?	**HSP (Henoch-Schonlein purpura)**
What is an important febrile illness that causes leukocytoclastic vasculitis?	**Kawasaki's disease**
What are some important general categories of things that cause leukocytoclastic vasculitis? (4 general categories)	1. Medications 2. Malignancy 3. Various infections/systemic diseases 4. Rheumatologic diseases
One clue that leukocytoclastic vasculitis is caused by SLE is the location of the lesions. What location is the clue?	**Vasculitis on the *digits***
Plaques over the knuckles, elbows, & knees, along with a heliotrope rash around the eyes = what diagnosis?	Dermatomyositis (the plaques are known as "Gottron's papules")
Plaques sometimes form on knuckles, knees, and elbows for patients with dermatomyositis. What other finding in the same areas goes along with juvenile dermatomyositis?	Calcinosis cutis (Calcifications in the skin over joints)
A picture of fingertips with a deeper red hue than usual near the lunula should be a tip-off to what rheumatological condition?	**Juvenile dermatomyositis** (the deeper red is dilated capillary loops)
Does sarcoid cause skin lesions?	Yes, often

What do the skin lesions of sarcoid look like?	Erythematous lesions often on the face – Especially nasal ala
It is often very difficult to differentiate sarcoid lesions from the lesions of what other disorder?	Discoid lupus lesions
Thickened, velvety, often darkened skin which is otherwise normal is called _____?	**Acanthosis nigricans**
Hyperinsulinism sometimes causes what change in the skin?	**Acanthosis nigricans**
Yellow, non-tender, noninflammatory superficial masses on the skin are called _____?	**Xanthomas**
Fatty deposits in the skin indicate what type of general medical problem?	**High cholesterol/ High triglycerides** (either one)
What is an "exanthem?"	Any skin eruption that occurs as a symptom of a general disease (exterior skin)
How is an "enanthem" different from an "exanthem?"	Enanthems are on *mucous membranes* (otherwise they are the same – Skin eruption as a symptom of a general disease)
Which gender is more likely to develop cutaneous drug eruptions?	Females
What situations tend to generate cutaneous drug reactions? (3 general situations)	• Multiple meds • Significant intercurrent disease (especially liver, renal, or connective tissue) • Viral illness while taking med

Where does the rash of a drug reaction usually start?

Trunk and proximal extremities

(spreads outwards in time)

What does a cutaneous drug reaction rash usually look like?

Maculopapular pink-red lesions (often become confluent)

Do bers form on the macules of a cutaneous drug eruption?

No, they should not (no vesicles, no pustules)

Does a cutaneous drug reaction indicate that your patient is at the beginning of a drug *hypersensitivity* syndrome?

Usually not

If a patient is going to develop a cutaneous drug eruption, how long into the drug therapy will they usually be when it begins?

1–2 weeks

(& it takes 1– 2 weeks to resolve)

What percentage of cutaneous drug reactions are the simple maculopapular type?

95 %

In addition to being maculopapular, what are other typical characteristics for a cutaneous drug reaction?

Itchy

&

Symmetrical lesions
(mainly morbilliform, meaning like measles – reddish macules, 2–10 mm each, sometimes confluent)

Which medication class most often causes cutaneous drug reactions?

β-Lactams

If a drug causes a cutaneous drug eruption, and the same drug is later given again, what sort of reaction is likely?

Either the same or increased reaction

What is a "complex" cutaneous drug reaction?

When it also has fever or other systemic symptoms

(cutaneous reaction by itself is called "simple")

How are cutaneous drug reactions appropriately treated?	Stop the drug & Supportive care
How can you differentiate the cutaneous drug reaction rash from a viral exanthem?	History & associated findings only
Which type of cutaneous drug reaction is second most likely, after the maculopapular type?	Urticarial (only 5 %)
Which type of cutaneous drug reaction is more commonly associated with fever and pruritis?	Urticaria
Which reaction typically develops faster, urticarial or maculopapular cutaneous drug reaction?	Urticarial – Develops in hours to days (Maculopapular requires 1–2 weeks)
What is the most common cause of urticaria in infants *less than* 6 months old?	**Cow's milk allergy**
Which age group of patients usually has the most dramatic appearing urticarial drug eruptions?	**Infants & young kids –** **Giant urticaria** & **Hemorrhagic urticaria**
Why would urticaria become hemorrhagic?	Leaky vessels → atraumatic hemorrhage
What are the most common drug causes of urticaria, in general? **(4 classes)**	**The usual suspects:** **1. Penicillins** **2. Tetracyclines** **3. Cephalosporins** **4. Sulfa drugs**
What is a "serum sickness-like reaction?"	**A reaction that looks the same as serum sickness, but immune complexes are not involved!**

Urticarial eruptions to penicillin are often due to _____? (type of reaction)	Type 1 (IgE)-mediated hypersensitivity
Opiates sometimes cause urticaria. What is the usual mechanism by which this occurs?	Mast cell degranulation
What causes serum sickness?	**Deposition of immune complexes in tissue**
Serum sickness has effects on many organ systems. What is its typical effect on the skin?	Usually urticarial
What usually causes serum sickness?	**Giving foreign proteins such as horse serum-based antivenoms or antithymocyte globulin made in rabbits**
What does a hemorrhagic urticarial lesion look like?	A bruise – Often the swelling (angioedema) is gone by the time the bruising appears
Which drugs are most often associated with the serum sickness-like reaction? (2)	**Cefaclor** & **Minocycline**
If urticarial drug reactions happen very quickly after beginning a medication, but maculopapular reactions require 1–2 weeks, how long does it usually take to develop serum sickness-like reaction?	**Usually 1–2 weeks**
Do antihistamines improve the symptoms of urticaria?	Yes
If serum sickness-like reaction is severe, how can you treat it?	Systemic steroids are helpful
What defines drug hypersensitivity *syndrome*? (not "reaction," but "syndrome")	**Internal organ involvement (+ rash + fever)**

Cutaneous findings in drug hypersensitivity syndrome vary a lot. What other clue on physical exam will help you to make the diagnosis?

Lymphadenopathy (usually diffuse)

Which general types of medications are most likely to trigger drug hypersensitivity syndrome?

Sulfa antibiotics

&

Anticonvulsants

Which anticonvulsants are especially likely to produce drug hypersensitivity syndrome? (& why is it important to know which ones?)

- **Phenytoin**
- **Phenobarbital**
- **Carbamazepine**

(all of these are "aromatic anticonvulsants")

– 80 % cross-reactivity among the group

If you stop an anticonvulsant that was causing a drug hypersensitivity syndrome, will the syndrome stop?

Usually – But it can continue to progress

If a drug is going to cause "hypersensitivity syndrome," how long after beginning the medication is it likely to start?

Less than 3 months

Can drug hypersensitivity syndrome produce toxic epidermal necrolysis (TEN) or Stevens-Johnson syndrome as its cutaneous manifestation?

Yes – But it usually causes generalized exfoliative erythroderma (any diffuse skin rash is possible)

In addition to the "aromatic anticonvulsants" which other anticonvulsant often causes cutaneous reactions?

Lamotrigine (Lamictal®) *15 % of kids on lamotrigine develop rash*

How often will lamotrigine produce a serious rash?

1 % of patients

How rapidly will a lamotrigine rash develop, after the medication is started?

First 2 months

What particularly concerning skin problem is unusually common with lamotrigine use?	Stevens-Johnson
Rashes with lamotrigine are most common in which patient group?	Children – 3× more common than in adults *(15 % of kids get a rash with lamotrigine)*
Lamotrigine is most likely to cause serious skin reactions when the dosing is done in what fashion? (2)	Unusually high initial dose Or Unusually fast escalation of dose
How is a "fixed drug eruption" defined? (4 components)	• Few lesions that do not move, on skin or mucosal surfaces • Lesions recur *at the same site* if the drug is reintroduced • Dusky color with some skin necrosis on histology • Hyperpigmentation after resolution
A diagnosis of Stevens-Johnson *requires* the involvement of how many mucous membranes?	*Two!*
Which usually comes first, the skin lesions or the mucosal lesions, in Stevens-Johnson?	**Mucosal lesions** (begin 1–2 days before skin lesions)
What comes before the skin or mucosal lesions in Stevens-Johnson?	Prodrome of systemic illness (fever, malaise, anorexia)
Which two mucous membranes are most often involved in Stevens-Johnson?	Eyes & mouth
Why must ophthalmology be consulted any time a patient develops Stevens-Johnson?	Pseudomembranes sometimes form & can cause permanent visual impairment (along with a variety of other possible complications, like corneal ulcers, eyelid problems, etc., which are also common in TEN)

Which one usually begins with discrete lesions that later coalesce – TEN or Stevens-Johnson?

Stevens-Johnson

How does TEN usually begin?

All-over sunburn (erythema)
then large bullae

How rapidly will Stevens-Johnson develop, in relation to when a medication was begun?

Within 2 months
(same timeline as usual for this type of disorder – TEN is the same)

In addition to the usual drug suspects, what other drug group sometimes causes TEN & Stevens-Johnson?

NSAIDs

Because TEN affects the skin diffusely, it can sometimes be confused with staph scalded skin syndrome. How can you differentiate them?

Staph scalded skin should *not* have mucous membrane involvement

How do you differentiate TEN & Stevens-Johnson based on the amount of body surface area affected?

<10 % is Stevens-Johnson

>30 % is TEN

(in between is considered an "overlap zone" & diagnosis depends on history)

Which is worse, TEN or Stevens-Johnson?

TEN

In addition to NSAIDs, which medication groups are most likely to produce TEN/Stevens-Johnson?

1. β-Lactams
2. Sulfa drugs
3. Aromatic anticonvulsants (phenobarb, phenytoin, carbamazepine)
4. Lamotrigine

Are the bers deeper in the skin layers in TEN or Stevens-Johnson?

They are the same!
(sorry to trick you)

What mortality is expected for pediatric TEN patients?

≤10 % with rapid treatment

(several series have no pediatric deaths – mortality is higher in adults)

**Who should care for TEN
or Stevens-Johnson patients?**

**A burn center –
Arrange rapid transfer**

**A patient with no significant (overall)
PMH is present with a generalized
erythematous rash which is now
developing some bullae. She recently
finished some ophthalmological
medications for a bacterial
conjunctivitis. She seems to be
systemically ill. What is her diagnosis?**

TEN in reaction to the ocular med
(probably a sulfa antibiotic)

**Which burn medication
is contraindicated for patients
with sulfa allergies?**

Silvadene™
(silver sulfadiazine)

Do the skin lesions of staph scalded
skin syndrome leave scars?

No –
It's subcorneal (within the dermis)

Where is the separation in the skin
in TEN & Stevens-Johnson syndrome?

Between the dermis and epidermis
(all of the epidermis comes off)

Which skin medication reactions
are supposed to be reported
(to the FDA & drug company)?

TEN
 &
Stevens-Johnson

Do TEN and Stevens-Johnson patients
have internal organ involvement from
these syndromes themselves?

No –
But they should be checked for this
because they may have had a drug
hypersensitivity syndrome
(organ reaction) *first!*

Are empiric antibiotics recommended
for TEN and Stevens-Johnson?

No

To the extent that we understand it,
why do some people develop TEN,
Stevens-Johnson, or drug hypersensitivity
syndrome?

Genetics –
Some people may not be able
to detoxify reactive metabolites

Will systemic steroids improve the
outcome in TEN?

No
(and they may increase infection rates)

What therapy has been found to be helpful in TEN?

IVIG

It is controversial whether erythema multiforme major is different from Stevens-Johnson. When is the term erythema multiforme major usually used?
   (3 criteria)

- Less generalized rash
- More inflammation & less necrosis
- Usually related to an infection rather than a drug

Do all three disorders, TEN, Stevens-Johnson, and erythema multiforme major include bering/bullae?

Yes

Which skin reaction disorder includes damage to internal organs?

Drug hypersensitivity syndrome

A child with fever, lymphadenopathy, and diffuse rash probably has a common infectious disease. What important cutaneous drug reaction *might* he or she have, though?

Drug hypersensitivity syndrome (treat with supportive, and steroids if organ involvement is severe)

How quickly will a drug hypersensitivity syndrome develop, after beginning the drug that causes it?

Usually within a few weeks (sometimes longer)

Which skin condition is a contraindication for smallpox vaccination?

Atopic dermatitis

(significantly more likely to have bad complications)

Pain on defecation, and erythema surrounding the anus, without any specific lesions, is often what diagnosis?

Perianal cellulitis (usually strep)

The "slapped cheeks" virus is _____?

Parvovirus B19

Human herpesvirus 6 is responsible for what very common childhood disease?

Roseola

Chapter 9
General Ophthalmology Question and Answer Items

What is strabismus?
When is strabismus normal, if ever?

Eye misalignment (crossed eye or deviated eye)
It is normal in the first few months of life, *if it is intermittent*

Is presbyopia a normal or abnormal finding?

Normal after age 40
(can't see well close-up)

What is presbyopia?

Lack of ability to accommodate that impairs near vision (caused by lens inflexibility, mainly)

What position does the eye end up in with a third cranial nerve palsy?

Down & out (like an intern)

(some prefer a third-year med student to remember CN3 – they're down & out because they're just getting started)

How does a cranial nerve 6 lesion present?

No lateral gaze (in the affected eye) –

Causes double vision & crossed eyes, depending on direction of gaze

What does a fourth cranial nerve palsy look like?
Why?

- Can't look down your nose! (you can't look down when your eye is medial – a fourth-year medical student can't look down his nose, because he or she isn't a doctor yet!)
- The superior oblique is paralyzed
  (their superiority muscle is paralyzed!)

© Springer Science+Business Media New York 2016
C.M. Houser, *Pediatric Tricky Topics, Volume 2*,
DOI 10.1007/978-1-4939-3109-5_9

Which autonomic system is responsible for constricting the pupil?

Parasympathetic

Mydriatics dilate the eyes. What class of medications do they generally belong to?

Sympathomimetics

What is the classic example of a mydriatic?

Atropine or homatropine (homatropine lasts up to *3 days,* and atropine *up to 2 weeks!)*

What is the medical term for constricting the pupil?

Miosis

What causes central retinal artery occlusion?

Usually emboli from the heart or carotid, but sometimes emboli that develop due to vasculitis

**How does central retinal artery occlusion present?
How is it treated?**

- **Sudden, painless, unilateral loss of vision**
- *Emergently!* **– must be treated within 90 min.**

You can try:
1. **Thrombolysis or pressure on the eyeball for a few seconds with sudden release (in an effort to move the obstruction)**
2. **Anterior chamber paracentesis (remove fluid to drop pressure suddenly – same idea as above)**
3. **Surgical intra-arterial thrombolysis**

What is the official name for a "stye?"

A hordeolum

What is the difference between a hordeolum and a chalazion?

- **Hordeolum – painful, red, at lid margin (a "whore" wearing red with painful lesions)**
- **Chalazion – painless lump, not at margin**

How are they treated?

Treatment is warm compresses (chalazions may sometimes be treated with I & D)

What is the main principle in treating chemical exposures of the eye?	Irrigate the heck out of it!! (confirm success with pH paper – you are done when the conjunctiva is at neutral pH)
Which is worse in the eye, acid or alkali? Why?	• Alkali • Acid burns, but alkali *melts* the cornea
What is preseptal cellulitis (also known as periorbital cellulitis)?	Infection of the skin and subcutaneous tissues *anterior* to the septal plate in the eyelid
How is orbital cellulitis different from preseptal or periorbital cellulitis?	It is still an infection of the soft tissues or the orbit, but posterior to the eyelid's septal plate
How common is loss of vision, in an eye with an orbital cellulitis infection?	Around 10 % is properly treated
What are the most common bugs to cause orbital cellulitis?	*With trauma history* – gram-negative rods *Without trauma history* – Staph & Strep bacteria + & H. flu type B (*H. flu* is less common now)
Which fungi are sometimes involved in orbital cellulitis, and mainly in which patient group?	Mucormycosis (faster course) & aspergillus (slower course) Immunocompromised patients
What are the most common bugs to cause preseptal (aka preorbital or periorbital) cellulitis?	Staph & Strep + H. influenza in children who are not immunized against it
How is herpes keratitis (corneal herpes) treated?	• Topical antivirals (meds that end in "idine") OR oral acyclovir (Cycloplegics are also used in some cases to reduce pain, as in other corneal disorders)
What is the associated buzzword?	• *Dendritic* keratitis (dendritic = looks like a tree on fluorescein exam)

In addition to topical antivirals and oral acyclovir, is there anything else you should do for a patient with herpes keratitis?

REFER TO OPHTHO!!!!!!!!

Patients with orbital cellulitis should always have what diagnostic performed, if possible?

CT to evaluate extent and location of infection and abscesses

How is orbital cellulitis treated?

Inpatient IV antibiotics

(surgical treatment is used only in certain cases, including failure to respond to antibiotic treatment)

What physical findings suggest orbital cellulitis?
(5)

1. *Restriction of eye movements*
2. *Proptosis*
3. **Decreased visual acuity**
4. **Severe pain on attempted eye movement**
5. **Afferent pupillary defect (Marcus Gunn pupil)**

(all signs need not be present)

What are the complications of orbital cellulitis?
(3)

Meningitis
Venous thrombosis
Blindness

(MVB, like MVP – in this case it's Most Valuable Bat, because you'll be blind as a bat with orbital cellulitis)

How is preseptal cellulitis treated?
What is proliferative diabetic retinopathy? When does this typically develop?

Outpatient antibiotics
- **New vessel growth on the retina**
- **Typically develops after many years of DM**

What are the typical changes of hypertensive retinopathy?
(5)

1. Arteriolar narrowing
2. Copper or silver wiring (vessel looks like wiring)
3. Cotton-wool spots (cotton-wool spots also go with CMV retinitis)
4. A-V nicking (arteriovenous nicking, like one vessel has squished the other a bit, when you see it through the ophthalmoscope)
5. Flame-shaped hemorrhages

Papilledema in a patient with hypertension (HTN) suggests what problem?

Hypertensive emergency
(the papilledema shows that the blood pressure is affecting the CNS, because the optic nerve is a cranial nerve)

Arteriolar narrowing, "copper wiring" of retinal vessels, and A-V nicking are all retinal signs of what systemic problem?

Hypertension
(Retinal arteries are narrow, or may have the appearance of "copper wires"
A-V nicking means that the vessels look acutely narrowed where they cross – as if the high-pressure artery "squished" the vein)

If a patient has hypertension, are there retinal signs of HTN that don't directly involve vessels?

Yes, but they are nonspecific

(cotton-wool spots & small hemorrhages)

What is glaucoma?
What are the two ways it occurs?
Which is more common?

- **Increased intraocular pressure**
- **Open angle and closed angle**
- **Open angle is *much* more common**

How is (regular) glaucoma treated?
(4)

Mainly with topical eye drops
1. β-Blockers (may have systemic effects)
2. α-Agonists
3. Sometimes acetazolamide or other carbonic anhydrase inhibitors
4. Sometimes surgery

(miotic agents like pilocarpine are also effective, but rarely used due to side effects)

How does regular (open-angle) glaucoma present?
(3)

1. Painless elevation of intraocular pressure
2. Enlargement of optic cup
3. Slow loss of visual field

Most commonly, cataracts in a neonate suggest what kind of general problem?

TORCH infection

T toxo & treponema
O other
R rubella
C cytomegalovirus
H herpes viruses

What is the most common cause of slow, painless, loss of vision?

Cataracts

What pediatric rheumatologic condition is commonly associated with uveitis?

Juvenile RA (rheumatoid arthritis)

What is UV keratitis?

Corneal inflammation due to ultraviolet exposure – looks like numerous tiny corneal abrasions on fluorescein exam

How do you get UV keratitis?

- **Welding**
- **Tanning (in a sunbed)**
- **Snow-skiing**

How do you treat a corneal abrasion of any type?
(4)

1. **Topical antibiotics (infection prevention)**
2. **Pain management (either PO, or a cycloplegic eye drop)**
3. **Tetanus immunization, if not up to date (an area of controversy – some do not give it)**

Is eye patching helpful for the comfort or healing of a corneal abrasion?

Generally not –
Patching should be avoided due to problems resulting from the patch, especially in kids <9 years old

Are there any situations in which you should prescribe steroid drops for the eyes?

NO
(Leave this to an ophthalmologist in your real-life practice,
&

don't **do it on the exam)**

What eye complications do you see with steroid use?
(2)

1. **Glaucoma**
2. **Cataracts**

    (topical, inhaled, and systemic steroids can all cause these)

What does a corneal ulcer with a "dendritic" pattern mean?

Herpes keratitis
(*big* deal – can cause blindness)

How can you tell whether someone is susceptible to an attack of acute angle-closure glaucoma?

Flat angles
(the cornea does not rise very steeply from the limbus, relative to the plane of the iris)

What are the two typical histories for someone presenting with angle-closure glaucoma?

1. **Just came from a dimly lit area (e.g., movie theater)**
2. **Anticholinergic medication use**

What are the hallmarks of viral conjunctivitis?
(3)

1. **Preauricular lymphadenopathy**
2. **Clear, watery discharge**
3. *Highly* **contagious**
   (healthcare workers, teachers, etc. should be quarantined for 14 days)

How does chlamydial conjunctivitis present?

Conjunctivitis *without* purulent discharge, 1–2 weeks after birth

(discharge may be mucoid, or just tear-like)

What are the signs of an acute angle-closure glaucoma attack?
(4)

1. Red eye
2. "hazy cornea" (due to water being forced into the corneal layers by the pressure)
3. Nausea & vomiting
4. Fixed and mid-dilated pupil *on one side only* (a trick reason for why a pupil might be "nonreactive" – it's stuck!)

In what situation might a patient be admitted to surgery for abdominal pain, then turn out to have an eye problem?

Acute angle-closure glaucoma (the abdominal effects of the rapidly increasing eye pressure can be quite impressive)

What is the main difference between the presentation of open-angle and closed-angle glaucoma, from the patient's perspective?

Closed angle is PAINFUL!

How is angle-closure glaucoma treated?

- Ophthalmology consult – *emergent*
- Temporarily, you can try pilocarpine, mannitol, glycerin, or acetazolamide
- Following pressure reduction – laser iridotomy (to give the fluid a permanent escape route)

What instrument is usually used to measure intraocular pressure?

A tonometer

Does conjunctivitis cause loss of vision?

By itself, no

What signs and symptoms go with allergic conjunctivitis?

Bilateral symptoms
Long duration
Itching
Watery discharge
Other allergy symptoms present (such as rhinorrhea)

How is viral conjunctivitis treated?

Supportive only

What is the most likely cause of conjunctivitis appearing in the first 24 h of life?
What is the likely causative agent?

- **Chemical conjunctivitis**
- **Silver nitrate drops given at birth (as a public health measure to prevent gonorrheal conjunctivitis)**

How do you treat gonorrheal conjunctivitis?	**Erythromycin ointment (parenteral third-generation cephalosporin treatment is also recommended for neonates)**
If a diagnosis or gonorrheal or chlamydial conjunctivitis is made, what additional steps must be taken for your patient & his or her family?	**Check for other sexually acquired diseases, if one has been identified (they often co-occur) Check Mom & partners for infection**
How does gonorrheal conjunctivitis present?	**Copious purulent discharge (2–5 days after birth, if it's neonatal)**
What is the order in which the three significant types of neonatal conjunctivitis present?	**1. Chemical 2. Gonococcal 3. Chlamydial** (clear, gunk, clear – like the discharge associated with each)
What is the hallmark of conjunctivitis?	Conjunctival injection (noticeably red vessels)
What is the most common cause of viral conjunctivitis?	**Adenovirus**
What treatment can be offered to patients with allergic (seasonal) conjunctivitis?	Cool compresses Artificial tears Antihistamine or mast cell stabilizer drops, if needed
What are the symptoms of central retinal vein occlusion? How is it treated?	• **Painless, unilateral, loss of vision over several hours** • **No treatment currently**
Which patients are most likely to develop central retinal vein occlusion ? (4)	Those with: 1. HTN 2. DM 3. Glaucoma 4. Hypercoagulable states

What buzzwords go with "retinal detachment?"

- **Flashes of light (at the edges of vision)**
- **Curtain or veil coming down**

Is retinal detachment painful?

No

Can retinal detachment be treated? If so, how?

Yes
The retina is reapposed via vitreoretinal surgery
(in the old days, or in low tech settings, the head was immobilized to allow gravity to reappose it)

Is retinal detachment an ophthalmological emergency?

No – you have at least 24 h to treat it
(it is an "urgency," but not something that must be seen immediately)

What are two rare causes of optic neuritis you should know?

- **Lyme disease**
- **Syphilis**

(both are treatable!)

How does optic neuritis present?

Painful, usually unilateral decrease in vision

Optic neuritis occurring in a young female = ?

Possible multiple sclerosis
(in real life, the correlation is not 100 % – the correlation is extremely high on the boards, however)

What type of optic neuritis can be painless?

Retrobulbar

Internuclear ophthalmoplegia (INO) on physical exam = what disease? Where is the lesion?

- MS (multiple sclerosis)
  (INO presents as inability to adduct the eye across midline, with nystagmus of the other eye on abduction)
- Medial longitudinal fasiculus (MLF of the brainstem)

What is the funduscopic appearance of optic neuritis?

Optic disc margins are blurred
(at least, on the boards they are – in real life, they may not be)

Optic neuritis in a male, with other neurological problems, suggests what general diagnosis?

Tumor

Bitemporal hemianopsia =

**A pituitary tumor
(as it grows upward, it compresses the optic chiasm)**

**A left homonymous hemianopsia
(both left visual fields are missing) = a lesion where?**

**Right optic tract
(after the chiasm)**

**A quadrantanopsia
(one quarter of the visual fields are missing) = a lesion where?**

**The optic radiations
(after the fibers split into an upper and lower group –
upper field radiations pass through the temporal lobe, lower through the parietal)**

Left homonymous hemianopsia *with macular sparing* = a lesion where?

Right occipital lobe

(It is not entirely clear WHY macular sparing at the cortical level occurs. Several theories exist, but the answer is not yet clear.)

Can strabismus be corrected later, after one eye no longer sees normally?

It can be corrected in childhood, but the younger the child the better the result is likely to be

Retinitis pigmentosa is sometimes presented on the photo section of the peds boards. What is it?

Degeneration of the photoreceptor cells in the retina – usually rods more than cones

How does a patient get retinitis pigmentosa?

**It is inherited
(Carrier state is common –
About 1:100 in US population)**

The inheritance pattern for retinitis pigmentosa is a little unusual – in what way?

All inheritance patterns are possible – there are many different mechanisms that cause RP

(autosomal dominant, autosomal recessive, and X-linked)

What is the classic presentation of retinitis pigmentosa?

Difficulty seeing in dim light environments, then . . . later "clumsiness" due to loss of peripheral vision (eventually producing tunnel vision)

What is esotropia?

Inward eye deviation

What is exotropia?

Outward eye deviation

Mnemonic:
"Ex" is for "external" deviation, away from the center of the body

What is the problem with not treating strabismus promptly?

Amblyopia will develop – (Permanent dyscoordination of gaze with poor vision in the deviating eye)

What is the "official" name for lazy eye?

Amblyopia

How is strabismus treated?

Three approaches:
1. Correct any refractive errors first
2. Patch the stronger eye for a few hours per day
3. Surgically correct extra-ocular muscle imbalance (less favored now)

What is pseudostrabismus or pseudoesotropia?

Eyes appear crossed inwards, due to prominent medial canthi (common in young babies, Asians, Down syndrome, etc.)

What is the simplest way to screen for strabismus?

Corneal light reflex
(If it's symmetric, there's no strabismus)

How are "cover tests" used to diagnose strabismus?

If gaze is conjugate, the eyes don't move once they fixate an object – even if one is covered

If there is strabismus, covering the fixated (straight) eye will cause the other eye to move (to gain fixation)

How bad does visual acuity have to be in children older than 5 years, to warrant an ophthalmology referral?	20/40 or worse in either eye (expected acuity is 20/20 at this age)
How bad does visual acuity have to be in very young children, age 3.5–5 years, to warrant an ophthalmology referral?	20/50 or worse in either eye (expected acuity 20/30 to 20/40)
Gonococcus is cultured on what type of medium?	**Thayer-Martin chocolate agar**
What will it say on micro, if conjunctivitis is caused by GC?	**Gram-negative *intracellular diplococci***
Can GC conjunctivitis be present at birth?	Yes, with premature rupture of membranes
If erythromycin prophylaxis is given, will it *prevent* neonatal chlamydial conjunctivitis?	*NO!* (although 14 days of *oral* erythromycin will cure it in 80 % of cases – the remainder will need a second course, but erythromycin is the preferred treatment)
***Intracytoplasmic inclusion bodies* are the buzzword for what infectious disease?**	**Chlamydia**
Erythromycin use in very young infants (<6 weeks old) increases the risk of what structural gut problem?	Pyloric stenosis
What is the long-term issue with chlamydial conjunctivitis?	**Corneal scarring**
Will *neonatal* chlamydial conjunctivitis cause corneal scarring?	No – it does in older individuals, but in neonates it's self-limited
Will neonatal gonorrheal conjunctivitis cause corneal scarring?	Yes – before silver nitrate was discovered, it was a leading cause of blindness

If an infant is determined to have either chlamydial or gonorrheal conjunctivitis, what must you evaluate?
(2 items)

- **Whether the Mom & partners have been treated**
- **Whether the infant has other STDs**

How do you treat a viral conjunctivitis?

Cool compresses/supportive care

What is the most common cause of viral conjunctivitis?

Adenovirus

What are the most common causes of bacterial conjunctivitis?
(4)

Staph
Strep
Moraxella
Hemophilus species

When is viral conjunctivitis most likely to occur?

Fall & winter

Do infants sometimes develop glaucoma?

Yes

What intraocular pressure suggests glaucoma in an infant?

>21 mm Hg

Which TORCH infection sometimes leads to infantile glaucoma?

Rubella

Which well-known genetic syndrome is most associated with glaucoma in infancy?

Sturge-Weber

How would an infant present with glaucoma?
(5 items – three are characteristics of the eye, three are effects found on exam)

1. **Enlarged cornea & eye**
   (known as "bulls eye" or buphthalmos)
2. **Cloudy cornea**
3. **Photophobia**
4. **Excessive tearing**
5. **Blepharospasm**
(meaning lid closure)

If a child has corneal enlargement due to glaucoma, what does that look like?

The affected eye is noticeably larger than the normal eye, and the cornea may be bluish or opaque

How can glaucoma in infants be treated?

1. **Laser surgery**
2. **β-Blocker ocular drops**
3. **Carbonic anhydrase inhibitor (ocular drops)**

(same as in adults)

What causes glaucoma, in general terms?

Failure to adequately drain the anterior chamber fluid

What two infectious diseases can sometimes cause a white pupillary reflex?

Toxocara & toxoplasmosis

In addition to retinoblastoma, what other retinal disorders can cause a white pupillary reflex?
(3)

Retinal detachment
Coats disease (a type of retinal detachment)
Retinal coloboma
(failure to fuse all portions of the eye – defect usually midline inferior)

What is Coats disease of the retina?

A disorder of retinal vessels that leads to serum leakage beneath the retina. The serum accumulation lifts and detaches the retina over time, and can cause a yellow or white retinal reflex

When genetic and metabolic disorders cause a white pupillary reflex, what is the usual reason?

Cataracts

How do you know which Sturge-Weber patient is most likely to develop infantile glaucoma?

If the "port-wine stain" involves V1 & V2 (eye & cheek) area, especially the eyelids, conjunctiva, or sclera

(bilateral port-wine stains also put the patient at increased risk)

Is "congenital glaucoma" typically present at birth?

Can be, but can develop later (weeks to months later)

For infants with primary glaucoma (high pressure <u>not</u> associated with any other disorder), how does that happen?

Multifactorial genetic misfortune

How long should you treat infantile glaucoma before consulting ophtho?

Consult them right away

(Risks are high, and medical therapy may not be enough)

Tearing in an otherwise well-appearing neonate is usually due to _____?

Nasolacrimal duct blockage/stenosis

What is nasolacrimal duct (NLD) blockage?

The NLD opens into both the medical edge of the eyelid and the nose, allowing it to drain tears into the nose (the reason your nose runs when you cry) If the opening into the nose is blocked or failed to open during development, tears cannot pass into the nose, causing excessive tearing from the eye

What is the recommended treatment for nasolacrimal duct stenosis or obstruction?

Massage & time
(Massage is supposed to move fluid and help to break up the offending membrane in the nose – it may just give parents something to do while time fixes the problem)

If an eye with nasolacrimal obstruction becomes infected, how is the infection treated?

Topical antibiotics & massage
(if not severe)

At what point should nasolacrimal duct obstruction be sent to ophthalmology?

Still there at 1 year

How is a *dacryocystocele* different from a blocked nasolacrimal duct?

In dacryocystocele, the fluid secreted in the lacrimal duct can't get out. There is a block at the puncti, the NLD opening at the eyelid AND a block in the nose opening. A cyst is therefore formed

In duct obstruction, tear fluid can't get into the lacrimal system → excessive tearing

What is the usual appearance of a dacryocystocele?

A small bulge, often with a bluish color, between the nose & the medial eye

What is the recommended treatment, from the pediatrician's perspective, of a dacryocystocele?

Rapid ophtho referral (the fluid in the cyst might get infected, and the infection can easily spread!)

If a dacryocystocele is infected, how should it be treated?

IV antibiotics & ophtho referral

Which has a mass associated with it – nasolacrimal duct stenosis, or dacryocystocele?

Dacryocystocele

(sometimes looks bluish)

If one eye is mechanically obstructed, and therefore cannot receive images in infancy or toddlerhood, what will happen?

The visual cortex will form without areas for that eye's input (cannot be fixed in adulthood & gets harder with increasing age in children!)

Why would a central retinal artery occlusion cause a "cherry red spot" on the retina?

Because the retina turns white without the retinal artery's blood supply, *except for the macula which has a dual blood supply*

How will the retina look with central retinal vein occlusion?

Too much blood – thick, tortuous vessels, optic nerve swelling & macular edema, some hemorrhage

If a patient has a chemical injury to the eye at home, should you advise them to irrigate it first, or transport for medical care first?

Irrigate – with A LOT of water

Why should a cycloplegic be given after a chemical injury to the eye?

1. Decreases the pain of ciliary muscle spasm
2. Reduces probability of adhesions between lens & iris

When should you limit your eye exam to basic acuity?

Globe rupture or corneal/scleral lacerations

If an eye trauma patient has crepitus in the vicinity of the eye, what has likely happened?

Paranasal sinus fracture (the open sinus is a risk for eye infection)

When trauma has occurred near the eye/orbit, which nerve's function is most likely to be compromised?

Infraorbital – test sensation on cheek beneath eyes, and upper lip/philtrum area

If you are concerned about a possible foreign body in the eye, but not globe rupture, what two components of your exam are critical?

Upper & lower lid eversion (to find it)
&
Fluorescein exam (to check the cornea for scratches)

A foreign body is especially likely to have penetrated the eye if your patient was exposed to what situation?

Metal on metal work

(pounding on metal with metal)

What is a hyphema?

Blood in the anterior chamber of the eye

What are the two main long-term complications of hyphema?

1. Glaucoma
2. Staining of the cornea

What special short-term worry must be dealt with in hyphema cases?

Risk of rebleeding – often occurs 3–5 days after the initial event

Why should cycloplegics be used in cases of hyphema?

Less movement in the anterior chamber means less chance of clot disruption

What are the symptoms of uveitis?

Pain
Photophobia
Decreased vision

What is an example of an ocular antihistamine that can be used in cases of allergic conjunctivitis?

Lodoxamide or olopatadine

An eyelid chalazion may take how long to resolve?

Six months

Can a chalazion be a chronic problem?

Yes, often is – when chronic it is a firm & painless mass

Which tumor is the most common metastatic tumor in the orbital area for children?

Neuroblastoma

(followed by Ewing sarcoma, Wilms tumor, and leukemia-related masses)

Metastatic neuroblastoma can have an unusual presentation when it occurs in the orbital area. What is it?	**Sudden onset of proptosis and bruising (can look like child abuse)**
What is the most common intraocular tumor in kids?	**Retinoblastoma**
What is the most common presentation of retinoblastoma?	**Leukocoria** **(meaning white retinal reflex)**
What common presentation of retinoblastoma results from the decreased vision in the eye?	**Strabismus –** **It is therefore important to check for the red reflex in all children presenting with strabismus** **(refer to ophthalmology for full evaluation)**
How is retinoblastoma acquired?	**Inherited:** **Autosomal dominant** (meaning that a germline mutation is present, and all body cells carry the altered gene) **Or** **Sporadic genetic mutation** (only the cells in the eye carry the gene)
Can both types of retinoblastoma inheritance types pass the tumor gene on to future generations?	**No – only the germline mutation can** (About 40 % of retinoblastoma patients have germline mutations. The remainder should not be at risk to pass the disorder on)
What proportion of retinoblastoma cases will be bilateral?	1/3
How is inherited retinoblastoma different from the sporadic type, in terms of its clinical consequences?	Inherited is more likely to be bilateral and multifocal There is also a risk of developing a pinealoma, an additional tumor type
Lens dislocation is a characteristic of which two genetic disorders?	**Marfan's** & **Homocystinuria**

In which direction does the lens dislocate in Marfan's?	**Up**
In which direction does the lens dislocate in homocystinuria?	**Like the IQ in homocystinuria – it goes** *down*
Does the feeling that a foreign body is in the eye go away when you remove the foreign body?	**Yes – if there's no corneal abrasion** **If there is an abrasion, the sensation will persist until the cornea heals**
What is iridodonesis, and what does it indicate?	**The iris trembles or wiggles easily, and it suggests the lens has dislocated** *(think of it as the free edge of the iris wiggling, because it is not supported by the lens anymore)*
A very sharp white optic disk and decreased vision =	**Optic atrophy**
What percentage of retinoblastoma patients will have a family history of retinoblastoma?	40 %
Most retinoblastoma patients present for treatment by what age?	Two years
What treatments are available for retinoblastoma?	**Chemotherapy** (systemic & intra-arterial) **Laser** **Cryotherapy** **Radiation therapy** **& Eye enucleation** (Radiation therapy is rarely used in this disorder, due to the increased chance of secondary tumors)
What percentage of "pink eye" is due to bacterial causes, versus viral causes?	>50 % bacterial
Can a patient develop herpes keratitis, without developing any skin lesions?	Yes

Has H. flu immunization changed the likely pathogens for orbital and periorbital cellulitis?	Yes – it's mainly staph and strep now
Contact lens wearers are at increased risk of what corneal problem?	Corneal ulceration (usually due to pseudomonas – needs ophtho consult now!)
Your patient loved the topic anesthetic drops you used to examine his corneal abrasion. Can you prescribe him some for home?	No – Increased risk of poor healing & new injury (can't feel surface of the eye, so it's not protected very well)
A patient presents with gradual unilateral decreasing vision, pain with eye movement, and field defects in the same eye's visual fields. What relatively common visual diagnosis is this likely to be?	Optic neuritis
What is blepharitis?	**Chronic inflammation/infection of the lid margins**
Is baby shampoo a good option for treating blepharitis?	**Yes – Sometimes topical antibiotics are also used**
What common skin disorder is blepharitis strongly associated with?	Seborrheic dermatitis
What is the triad of classic Horner syndrome?	**Ptosis Miosis Anhidrosis (no sweating on affected side)**
What causes Horner syndrome?	**Damage to the sympathetic chain (at various points)**
What three medications can be used to treat CMV retinitis, seen in immunocompromised patients?	Valganciclovir Foscarnet & Cidofovir

What is the usual pathophysiology of retinopathy of prematurity (ROP)? (3 steps)	1. High-concentration $O_2 \rightarrow$ retinal vasoconstriction 2. Retinal capillaries are damaged 3. Retinal vessels proliferate in response
Some premature infants are at risk for retinopathy of prematurity (ROP) only if exposed to high oxygen levels. What defines this group?	30–35 weeks' gestation & Birth weight between 1300 & 1800 g
Which premature neonates are <u>always</u> at risk for ROP?	<30 weeks' gestation Or <1300 g *(even if there is no supplemental oxygen exposure)*
When should infants be routinely assessed for the presence of ROP?	At discharge, or when they reach 4 weeks old – whichever comes first
If an infant has known ROP, how often should ophthalmology reevaluate his/her retinas?	Every 1–2 weeks (depending on severity)
What does "plus disease" of ROP refer to?	Tortuous & engorged blood vessels near the optic disk
When can frequent ophthalmology evaluations of ROP retinas be discontinued?	**When the retina is fully vascularized**
When intervention is necessary, how is retinopathy of prematurity treated?	Laser therapy (if untreated when laser was indicated, 50 % will develop blindness in the affected eye)
As increasing amounts of fibroproliferative matter forms on the retina in ROP, what mechanical problem can develop?	**Retinal detachment** **(stage 4 disease)**
What causes a white papillary reflex in a neonate? (4 options)	1. **Retinoblastoma** 2. **ROP (retinopathy of prematurity)** 3. **Retinal coloboma** 4. **Cataracts**

Chapter 10
General Ear, Nose, and Throat
Question and Answer Items

If a child has otorrhea from the myringotomy tubes, what should you do?	Topical antibiotic eardrops have high efficacy, although unusual organisms are more common for kids with tubes than for those without
How can you remember which test is the Rinne, and which is the Weber?	WEBER has two "Es" so it's between the ears (the tuning fork is held at the vertex of the forehead – should hear it equally)
How is the Rinne test performed?	Tuning fork on the mastoid, then beside the ear, in the air – Air should be heard better (still heard after the mastoid is silent)
"Sudden" hearing loss is defined as loss of hearing that occurs over 3 days or less. What are four conduction problems that can cause sudden hearing loss?	**1. Cerumen impaction (most common)** **2. Foreign body** **3. TM or ossicle problems** **4. Middle ear fluid**
When performing a hearing exam, how does bilateral sensorineural hearing loss present?	Bilaterally decreased hearing with normal Weber & Rinne

© Springer Science+Business Media New York 2016
C.M. Houser, *Pediatric Tricky Topics, Volume 2*,
DOI 10.1007/978-1-4939-3109-5_10

Which medical conditions predispose the patient to sudden sensorineural hearing loss? (4)	**1. DM** **2. Hyperlipidemia** **3. Vascular hypercoagulable states** **4. Meniere**
What is a typical environmental cause of sudden sensorineural hearing loss?	Noise
What is a likely infectious cause of sudden sensorineural hearing loss (general category)?	Viruses (especially mumps, in unimmunized kids)
What is a likely cause of sudden sensorineural hearing loss in a hospitalized patient?	Medication
Do tumors cause sudden sensorineural hearing loss?	Yes – Especially if there is a small associated hemorrhage
Which medications are most notorious for causing sensorineural hearing loss? (5 categories)	**1. Loop diuretics (especially ethacrynic acid)** **2. NSAIDs** **3. Salicylates** **4. Certain antibiotics (e.g., gentamicin)** **5. Chemo regimens**
It's sad if you lose your hearing. How can the mnemonic "SAD" help you remember the drugs most likely to cause this problem?	**SAD CHEMicals** **Salicylates (& NSAIDs)** **Antibiotics (& alcohol)** **Diuretics (loop)** **CHEMicals (reminds you of chemo regimens)**
When a patient complains of headache or ear pain, what source of the pain should always be considered?	**Tooth pain**
Why is perichondritis a worrisome infection?	**The infection rapidly damages the underlying cartilage –** **Cosmetic result is bad**

Where is perichondritis most often seen?	**Pinna of the ear**
What unusual infectious agents must you watch for perichondritis? (2)	**Pseudomonas** & **Proteus**
Which bacterium is most often identified in otitis externa?	**Pseudomonas (60 %)**
Is a TM perforation an ENT emergency?	**No –** **Follow-up with ENT later that week**
What percentage of TM perforations heals spontaneously?	**90 %**
What are the most typical or widely cited causes for TM perforation? (4)	1. Noise 2. Barotrauma 3. *Blunt* or penetrating trauma 4. Lightning strike (especially if the patient is found undressed or in arrest)
What is the hallmark of otitis externa on exam?	**Pain with movement of the pinna**
What is a feared complication of otitis externa?	**Malignant otitis externa**
Which patients are likely to develop malignant otitis externa?	**Diabetics – 90 % of patients are diabetic** **(other immunodeficient patients are also at increased risk)**
What is the "triad" of Meniere disease?	**1. Vertigo** **2. Tinnitus** **3. Sensorineural hearing loss** (to reduce recurrences low-salt diet & hydrochlorothiazide may be helpful)
What other patient group presents similarly to Meniere patients?	**CPA tumor** **(cerebellopontine angle)**

What is the natural history of Meniere disease?

Intermittent recurring attacks that last weeks to years (treatment doesn't work well, but is improving)

Most treatments for Meniere disease focus on what aspect of the auditory system?

Reducing pressure in the endolymphatic portion of the affected ear

What differentiates labyrinthitis from vestibular neuronitis?

Labyrinthitis includes *hearing loss!*

(not just vertigo or tinnitus)

What is the most common cause of peripheral vertigo?

Benign positional vertigo (BPV)

What are the typical features of BPV, in terms of the patients' movement or position?

- **Worse in certain positions**
- **Worse with head motion**

What is the typical onset for BPV?

Gradual

What is the natural course of BPV?

Spontaneous resolution

What "key" should you find on physical exam, if you are able to elicit the vertigo of BPV?

Fatiguing (horizontal) nystagmus

(fatiguing means that it decreases, then stops, on its own)

What are the most concerning complications of sinusitis?
(4)

1. **Cavernous sinus thrombosis**
2. **Pott's puffy tumor (skull osteomyelitis on the forehead)**
3. **Orbital cellulitis**
4. **Brain abscess**

Sinusitis has the same typical bacterial pathogens as which other ENT infection?

What are the pathogens?

- **Otitis media**
- **Strep pneumo**
- **H. flu (non-typeable)**
- **M. catarrhalis**
- **Anaerobes (especially with chronic infection)**

(S. pyogenes is also a common cause of otitis media, but not common in sinusitis)

What is "ring sign" supposed to tell you?	**Whether fluid dripping from the nose is snot or CSF**
	(a ring should form around a droplet on filter paper if it's CSF – but it's very unreliable in reality)
Why is a septal hematoma (in the nose) a big deal?	**Because without rapid treatment the pressure causes septal necrosis –**
	"saddle nose" **deformity results**
Where do most nosebleeds come from?	**Anterior veins of the nose (along the septum)**
(give two names for it)	**Or**
	Kiesselbach's plexus (same thing)
Patients with posterior epistaxis make up what percentage of epistaxis patients overall?	**5 %**
	(fortunately)
What is the biggest risk factor for posterior epistaxis?	Arteriosclerosis
What are the main risks involved in posterior epistaxis? **(2)**	1. **Hypovolemia** 2. **Aspiration**
How is posterior epistaxis treated?	**Posterior nasal pack**
What must you watch out for with patients who have a posterior nasal pack? **(4)**	1. **Hypoxia & CO_2 retention (due to airway obstruction)** 2. **Bradycardia (vagal response)** 3. **Sinusitis/OM** 4. **Coronary ischemia (due to stress and hypovolemia, in a patient at risk for ischemia)**
What is the correct disposition for a patient with posterior epistaxis who has had a posterior pack placed?	**Admit to ICU for observation under ENT's supervision**

In cavernous sinus thrombosis, which cranial nerves are likely to be affected?

Ipsilateral 3, 4, 5, & 6 –

CN6 is usually the FIRST affected, because it is not well anchored compared to the other two, so it is most easily stretched by the increasing pressure

Which infections are likely to produce cavernous sinus thrombosis?

Midface infections –

Sinusitis, periorbital cellulitis, dental

Who was LeFort?

A guy who dropped cadavers from heights to find out how their faces would fracture

How did LeFort classify facial fractures?

Three groups:
LeFort 1 – the maxilla moves freely
LeFort 2 – the maxilla & nose move freely
LeFort 3 – the maxilla, nose, & cheeks (to the orbits) move freely

(in other words, the *whole* midface is mobile as a unit)

Why is a LeFort facial fracture concerning?
(3)

1. *Risk of airway compromise* (teeth or bleeding in airway)
2. Risk of basilar skull fracture or associated c-spine injury
3. Risk of brain injury
4. Risk of tooth malocclusion if not properly repaired

What is the most common complication of outpatient ENT surgery?

Post-op hemorrhage

Historically, what was the most common cause of epiglottitis?

H. flu

Which vessel is the most common culprit in posterior epistaxis?

The lateral nasal branch of the *sphenopalatine artery*

How does chronic otitis media spread to other locations?

It erodes nearby bone

What is the most common cause of sialadenitis worldwide?

Mumps

Excruciating stabbing or electric shock-type pain to the cheek with sudden onset, that waxes & wanes, typically in a female patient =

Tic Douloureux (trigeminal neuralgia)

If there is a hematoma on the pinna, how should it be treated and why?

- **It must be aspirated (evacuated) then dressed with a pressure dressing to prevent it from refilling**
- **Without treatment the cartilage deforms and causes cauliflower ear**

A hard, rounded swelling of the hard palate or posterior mandible that is not tender is likely to be what diagnosis?

Torus palatinus/torus mandibularis

What is trench mouth, and what organism causes it?

- Acute necrotizing ulcerative gingivitis
- Treponema vincentii

Mnemonic:
Think of *Vincent* van Gogh with bad teeth to remember the organism

How is trench mouth treated?

Metronidazole
&
Penicillin

(surgical debridement may also be needed)

What is the typical age group for croup?

6 months to 6 years
(typically <3 years)

What is the other name for croup?

Laryngotracheobronchitis

What infection produces "lumpy jaw syndrome?"

Actinomycosis (the one with "sulphur-colored crystals")

(Remember that a single lump on the jaw of an African child is usually Burkitt's lymphoma)

What are the most important risk factors for rhinocerebral mucormycosis?

Neutropenia
&
Diabetic ketoacidosis

A child presents with ear pain and fluid-filled blisters on the tympanic membrane. What is the *most likely* diagnosis and its associated organism?

- **Bullous myringitis**
- **Mycoplasma is most associated in the literature BUT the typical otitis media pathogens are actually more common**

What diagnosis and related organism should always be considered in a child who seems to have bullous myringitis?

- **Ramsay-Hunt**
- **Herpes**

The main treatment for rhinocerebral mucormycosis is . . .?

Surgical debridement (+ antifungals IV)

High mortality!

Where do preauricular sinus tracts come from?

Failure of the first & second branchial arches to fuse properly

Why must nasal packing be removed promptly (24–48 h) after placement?

Toxic shock syndrome can develop!

(The antibiotics prescribed to prevent sinusitis while the packing is in are somewhat preventative)

Which laryngeal ring is essential in airway patency?

The cricoid (goes the whole way around)

Which sinuses are present at birth?

**Sphenoid
Ethmoid (one or two cells)
Maxillary**

(sources differ on the ethmoid – some say it is present, others dispute that)

What is the diagnostic test of choice for neck masses?

FNA
(fine-needle aspiration)

Does anticoagulant therapy improve outcome in patients with cavernous sinus thrombosis?

No

What study is preferred to diagnose cavernous sinus thrombosis?	CT or MRI
What is the most common organism found in retropharyngeal abscesses?	β-Hemolytic strep
At what age does retropharyngeal abscess typically occur?	6 months to 3 years
How does retropharyngeal abscess present?	Fever Ill to toxic appearing Stridor Dysphagia +/− Drooling Refusal to eat Little movement (it hurts)
What is the most feared complication of lateral pharyngeal space infections?	Septic thrombophlebitis of the jugular vein *(Lemierre's syndrome)*
What is the usual bacterial agent in Lemierre's syndrome?	Fusobacterium (others are possible, and is often polymicrobial)
A teenager presents with a sore throat, but seems genuinely ill, with fever & rigors. What serious disorder should you consider?	Lemierre's syndrome
What is the most common congenital laryngeal disorder?	Laryngomalacia
If a mandibular tumor has a "soap-bubble" appearance on X-ray, what is it?	Ameloblastoma
What three signs should you look for on physical exam when evaluating for basilar skull fracture?	1. Blood behind the TM (hemotympanum) 2. Raccoon eyes 3. Battle's sign (bruising over the mastoid)

What two presenting complaints are most common with acoustic neuromas?

1. **Hearing loss**
2. **Tinnitus**

What is the most common laryngeal tumor of children?

Laryngeal papillomas

Which major artery runs through the cavernous sinus?

The internal carotid

**Adolescent male +
nose bleed +
nasal obstruction =**

Juvenile nasopharyngeal angiofibroma

What is the most characteristic finding on physical exam of a patient with malignant otitis externa?

Granulation tissue in the external auditory meatus

Diplopia after facial trauma suggests what diagnosis?

Orbital floor fracture

A patient presents with fever, malaise, and a dark red raised lesion – painful to touch – on his face. The lesion is expanding over time. What is the likely diagnosis?

Erysipelas

Only one muscle abducts the vocal cords. Which one?

Posterior cricoarytenoid

Infection and edema spreading from the lower part of the oral cavity into the neck is called . . .?

Ludwig's angina –

Neck is usually described as having "brawny edema"

What usually gets Ludwig's angina started?

Dental work

Technically, what is Ludwig's angina, and why is it called "angina?"

- **Bilateral submandibular cellulitis**
- **"Angina" just means "pain" (not specific to the heart)**

What types of organisms are usually involved in Ludwig's angina?	Mixed aerobic & anaerobic
If an item mentions "brawny edema" of the anterior neck, what diagnosis should you be thinking of?	Ludwig's angina *(Brawny just refers to the skin color deepening due to underlying infection)*
What is the most common cause of death in Ludwig's angina?	Airway obstruction
Can a dermoid cyst be found in the mouth?	Yes – Along the floor of the mouth
What is the diagnostic test of choice for acoustic neuromas?	MRI with gadolinium contrast
In general, how can you differentiate viral sialadenitis from bacterial sialadenitis?	Viral – usually bilateral Bacterial – usually unilateral
What two important structures are often injured by horizontal (ear to lip) cheek lacerations?	The parotid duct & Facial nerve
What noninfectious cause of salivary gland problems should you be aware of?	Calculi – They sometimes block salivary outflow
What is one clue that your patient's salivary gland problem is caused by obstruction?	Symptoms get worse with induction of salivation – Sometimes this also pushes the calculous out *(Give them some lemon to suck on!)*
How can you remember which duct comes from the parotid gland, and which from the submandibular?	Parotid – <u>S</u>tensen's is from the <u>S</u>ide Submandibular – Wharton's. W looks like the floor of the mouth, looking straight on at it
What two causes of gingival hyperplasia are important to remember?	1. Phenytoin 2. Acute leukemia

How do you treat acute necrotizing ulcerative gingivitis?

Metronidazole
&
Penicillin

(Surgical debridement is often also necessary)

What is the most common deep infection of the head and neck, and which age group tends to get it?

Peritonsillar abscess –
Young adults & adolescents

Aside from the patient's discomfort, what is the most concerning aspect of a peritonsillar abscess?

Spread to the adjacent tissue planes producing
1. Serious infection
2. Airway compromise

What is the buzzword for peritonsillar abscess findings on physical exam?

Uvula deviation
(away from the abscess)

What is bacterial tracheitis?

Bacterial infection of the interior trachea –
Usually staph

Which patient group is at greatest risk to develop bacterial tracheitis?

People who have had their tracheas manipulated

(especially those with tracheostomies in place)

Why is bacterial tracheitis concerning?

1. Very toxic infection
2. Copious secretions can compromise the airway

Rapid onset of a *very sore throat, fever,* & no findings on oropharyngeal exam, +/– stridor = what diagnosis?

Epiglottitis

Lateral neck X-ray shows a "thumb print" – what is the diagnosis?

Epiglottitis

What is the treatment for significant croup?

1. Inhaled racemic epinephrine
2. Steroids

(2)

What must you watch out for, if a child has received racemic inhaled epinephrine, as a treatment for significant croup?

Rebound of symptoms when the epinephrine wears off – a dose of steroid given early in treatment should help to prevent this

(about 3 h of observation is usually recommended)

If you suspect epiglottitis, what must you *not do?*

DO NOT try to visualize the epiglottis or stick anything in the mouth

(risk of closing off the airway)

What is trismus?

Difficulty opening the jaw

How can you remember the causes of trismus (mnemonic)?

It would be hard to kiss on a DATE with trismus:

Dystonia
Abscess
Tetanus
Epiglottitis

(Abscess could be peritonsillar, retropharyngeal, Ludwig's angina, etc.)

How can you tell a thyroglossal cyst from a branchial cleft cyst on physical exam?

Thyroglossal are central
(between the thyroid & tongue)

Branchial are lateral

Mnemonic:
Branches grow laterally!

What is the buzzword for trigeminal neuralgia?

"Electric shock" facial pain

What medication is often used for the pain of trigeminal neuralgia?

Carbamazepine

How is leukoplakia different from candida on physical exam?

Leukoplakia *cannot be scraped off* and is *not painful*

Which patients are likely to develop oral leukoplakia?
(3 groups)

Smokers
Males
Immunocompromised

Does leukoplakia develop into cancer?

Sometimes

How is leukoplakia associated with trauma?

Local trauma sometimes seems to get it started

Nasal polyps in a child <12 years old should make you suspect what diagnosis?

**CF
(In older kids, it's more likely to be associated with allergic rhinitis)**

It would seem reasonable to treat nasal polyps with decongestants to decrease their size. Have decongestants been effective for polyp treatment?

No

What medications have been shown to be very effective in decreasing the size of nasal polyps – especially for CF patients?

Steroids

What infectious disease predisposes to development of nasal polyps?

Chronic sinusitis

Other than being annoying, can nasal polyps cause real problems?

Yes –
Can sometimes obstruct or even *deform the nose*

If nasal polyps require treatment, what can be done?

Surgical removal
(but they often grow back for CF patients)

What is the most common cause of epistaxis in children?

Nose picking!

(Discreetly put, and so that you can recognize it on an exam, "local digitally induced trauma")

To remove a foreign body in the office of ER setting, what equipment/meds are needed?
(4 items: 2 meds, 2 equipment)

1. Topical anesthetic (e.g., viscous lidocaine)
2. Vasoconstrictor (e.g., neosynephrine)
3. Forceps
4. Suction

An adolescent presents with anterior epistaxis – what should you remember to ask him or her?

"Are you using cocaine?"

(It irritates, and can even eat through, the nasal septum – due to its strong vasoconstrictive properties)

What do nasal polyps look like?

Gray, grapelike masses

What is the most common congenital anomaly of the nose?

Choanal atresia

After surgical correction, what common complication develops for many choanal atresia patients?

Restenosis

If only one side is affected by choanal atresia, what should be done?

Surgical repair – but you can wait a few years to do it

Anytime you diagnose a child with choanal atresia, what else should you be looking for?

The CHARGE abnormalities –

Coloboma
Heart problems
Atresia (choanal)
Retarded growth & intellect
Genital anomalies
Ear problems/deafness

What is "lingual ankyloglossia?"

When the frenulum under the tongue limits its anterior movement significantly ("tongue tied")

Why is lingual ankyloglossia a problem for some newborns?

If the tongue can't get past the alveolar ridge, breast feeding is difficult

What social activity is potentially a big problem for the lingual ankyloglossia patient?

Licking an ice cream cone

If treatment for lingual ankyloglossia is desired, what is done?

Snip the frenulum (frenulectomy) in the office

Thyroglossal cysts are usually asymptomatic. Why might you be worried about one?

When infected, they can rapidly expand & compromise the airway

What is the management of thyroglossal duct cysts?

Surgical excision

If a child is described as having a "divided" or "lobulated" tongue, what should you expect to find on the rest of physical exam?

- Lip & palate issues
- Digit issues
- Usually part of an overall syndrome

Should lab tests be ordered for children who appear to have URIs?

No

Which viruses typically cause URIs?

Rhinoviruses
&
Coronaviruses

(+ adenoviruses, enteroviruses, influenza, & parainfluenza, among others)

What is the significance of thick green or yellow nasal discharge in the first week of an apparent URI?

None –
It *does not* indicate sinusitis

Are antihistamines helpful when treating URIs?

No –
Actually harmful as they decrease mucous clearance

If a school-aged child has a URI, and then gets worse with a new fever, sore throat, & cough about 10 days into the illness, what is the diagnosis?

Sinusitis

How does sinusitis present in school-aged kids?

Fever
Nasal discharge
Cough – especially at night

How does sinusitis present in adolescents/adults?

Headache
Fever
Facial pain & tenderness

Is it helpful to take a nasal swab culture to identify the organism causing sinusitis?	**No – Useless**
If a possible sinusitis patient is also severely immunocompromised, what is the most certain way to diagnose it and ensure appropriate treatment?	**Aspirate the sinus directly via the face (!)**
Aspirating a sinus would be acceptable in which patient populations?	**1. Severe immunocompromise 2. Life-threatening illness 3. Not responding to therapy**
What is "Pott's puffy tumor?"	**Osteomyelitis/abscess of the frontal bone** **(generally due to frontal sinusitis)**
What is the most common *bacterial* cause of acute pharyngitis?	**Strep pyogenes (Group A)**
What percentage of all acute pharyngitis is due to strep pyogenes?	**15 %** **(It's almost all *viral!*)**
A sexually active adolescent with pharyngitis might have what type of pharyngitis?	**Gonococcal pharyngitis (yikes!)**
Exudates on the tonsils strongly suggest a bacterial cause for pharyngitis. True or false?	False
What symptom/sign constellation *does* suggest a bacterial cause for pharyngitis?	• **Diffuse erythema of tonsils & pillars** • **Soft palate petechiae** • **No other URI symptoms**
Coryza, long-lasting fever, postnasal discharge, pharyngitis, tender cervical lymphadenopathy, and anorexia in a child less than 2 years old is known as _____?	**Streptococcosis (Can last 8 weeks!)**

How long do we have *to start antibiotics* for strep throat, if the goal is to avoid rheumatic heart disease?	Nine days
How long is a strep throat patient contagious, after antibiotic therapy is begun?	Only a few hours (can go to school/daycare 24 h after treatment begins)
Which patients may have a prolonged course of sore throat, accompanied by numerous coryza symptoms, due to streptococcus?	Those <2 years old (can last 8 weeks – streptococcosis)
Although epiglottitis is much less common these days due to immunization, what is the most common cause when it does occur in pediatric patients?	*H. flu* (still!) – Followed by staph & strep species
When epiglottitis occurs in adolescents or adults, what are the usual pathogens (in general terms)?	Polymicrobial
Tonsillectomy used to be wildly popular. When is it currently recommended?	1. If needed to exclude tumor 2. Severe obstructive sleep apnea 3. Severe adenoidal/tonsillar hypertrophy 4. Recurrent pharyngitis (also may be recommended for recurrent otitis media)
What qualifies as "recurrent pharyngitis," as an indication for tonsillectomy?	• Three episodes each year for 3 years • Five episodes each year for 2 years • Seven episodes in 1 year
Does tonsillectomy decrease URIs?	No
Will tonsillectomy decrease the likelihood of chronic otitis media?	No
Does tonsillectomy decrease sinus infections – either acute or chronic?	No

Does adenoidectomy decrease the likelihood of recurrent or chronic otitis media, if the adenoids are hypertrophied?

Yes

(It is an indication for adenoidectomy)

Can persistent mouth breathing be an indication for adenoidectomy?

Yes

(The palate can actually deform due to persistent mouth breathing!)

Can persistent or frequent nasopharyngitis be an indication for adenoidectomy?

Yes, if the infections correlate with times that the adenoids were particularly hypertrophied

What is the most common cause of bacterial tracheitis?

Staph aureus

When bacterial tracheitis occurs in otherwise normal children (no neck or airway problems prior to infection), how is it usually managed?

- Admit (usually about 2 weeks)
- Intubate
- IV antibiotics (e.g., ceftriaxone, with nafcillin)

Which patients are most likely to develop bacterial tracheitis?

- **Patients with instrumented airways**
- **<3 years old**

High fever, brassy cough, and stridor in a young child are a likely presentation for which two diagnoses _____?

Croup
   Or
Bacterial tracheitis

How can you differentiate croup from bacterial tracheitis?

Bacterial tracheitis –

Patient is sicker & doesn't respond to croup measures (e.g., cool air, racemic epinephrine)

What causes inspiratory stridor (what is the mechanism)?

Partial obstruction *at or above the larynx*

Is stridor common in newborns?

Yes –
The airway is very narrow anyway, so stridor often develops before age 2 years

"Wet" sounding or *variably pitched* inspiratory stridor indicates that the source of the problem is _____?

Laryngomalacia
(the most common cause of inspiratory stridor)

If a patient's stridor is *worse when lying down*, and *improves with expiration*, what is it likely to be caused by?	**Laryngomalacia**
A neonate whose stridor *worsens when he or she is agitated* probably has what underlying problem?	**Laryngomalacia**
***High-pitched* inspiratory stridor in an infant with a *weak cry* is typically due to _____?**	**Vocal cord paralysis**
Why might an infant have a paralyzed vocal cord? (2 reasons)	1. Birth trauma to the recurrent laryngeal 2. CNS problem (various sorts)
What is another laryngeal reason that a neonate might have a weak cry?	**Laryngeal web**
How much can the tympanogram tell you about how well the child is hearing?	**Nothing –** **It measures the movement of the TM** **(The kid could have a perfect tympanogram, but have sensorineural deafness)**
When tympanograms are presented on the boards, what do they usually show?	Normal findings Or Poor technique
If a tympanogram is flat, what does that tell you?	**Poor mobility –** **The TM is stiff, or fluid is pushing against it**
If your patient with tympanostomy tubes in place get a tympanogram, and it is low amplitude (flat), how should you interpret that?	**The tubes are blocked**
If the tympanogram is unusually high, what does that mean?	**Hypermobile TM**

What is the significance of the area-under-the-curve for tympanography?	**It is a measure of the volume of the external auditory meatus**
If there is a TM perforation, what will the tympanogram show?	**Large area under the curve (because the canal is open to the middle ear)**
What would you expect to see for the area-under-the-curve on a tympanogram for a patient with myringotomy tubes that are functioning properly?	Large area under the curve (the EAM is open to the tube)
Postauricular swelling and erythema, especially if the pinna is pushed out from the head, suggest what infectious disease diagnosis?	**Mastoiditis**
How is mastoiditis treated?	Surgery & IV antibiotics
What infant feeding position increases the child's probability of developing otitis media?	**Horizontal positioning – child lying flat**
If the TM is erythematous, and you suspect OM from history, can you make the diagnosis?	No – Not enough physical findings
Are antihistamines or decongestants helpful for treating OM?	No
Are antihistamines or decongestants helpful in preventing OM?	No
When is it reasonable to change your antibiotics regimen for OM?	**After 3 days of PO treatment, if fever or pain continues**
In addition to "nose picking," what other situation often precipitates anterior epistaxis?	Dry air (for example, wintertime heating)

A developmentally delayed child presents with otorrhea, and pain with pinna movement. Diagnosis?
   (2 options)

- Foreign body
- Otitis externa

Will decongestants or antihistamines help in cases of middle ear effusions?

No

Why can a middle ear effusion be such a big deal?

It can decrease hearing (conductive hearing loss), which delays speech & language development

If middle ear fluid is present for more than 3 months, and the child has not had antibiotic treatment, what is the next step in management?

Evaluate for hearing loss – if <20 dB loss compared with expected hearing level, repeat testing after a further 3–6 months (earlier if there are signs of a possible problem)

In which patients with persistent middle-ear effusion should you consider more aggressive management, according to guidelines?

Those already "at risk" for developmental, speech & language problems –

e.g., other sensory impairments, autism, craniofacial disorders, or existing developmental disorder

What percentage of children with middle-ear effusion lasting 3 months will spontaneously clear that infection, over 12 months?

Only 30 %
(so significant follow-up testing for adequate hearing will be needed)

At what point should you stop watchful waiting (with regular interval hearing examinations) for a patient with a middle-ear effusion?

1. **Effusion has resolved**
2. **Hearing loss is identified**
3. **Structural abnormalities are suspected**

If the hearing evaluation indicates a loss of 21–40 dB, what does that mean for management?

It is a relative, but not absolute, indication for myringotomy tube placement

At what level of hearing loss is further management absolutely indicated?

40 dB

If a middle-ear effusion meets criteria for treatment, what is the recommended treatment for most patients?

Bilateral myringotomy with pressure equalization tube placement

Chronic bacterial infection of the middle ear is called _____?

Chronic suppurative otitis media

Chronic suppurative otitis means that a bacterial infection has continued for more than 6 weeks, despite treatment. What ear complication is this condition especially likely to produce?

Cholesteatoma

Can environmental factors cause middle ear effusions? If so, give some examples.

Yes, due to inflammation of the eustachian tube

- Smoke
- Allergens
- Infection

Which kids are most likely to develop acute otitis media with resistant strains of Strep pneumo?
(3)

1. <2 years old
2. In daycare
3. Received antibiotics in past month

Most acute otitis media is caused by which two organisms, if it is bacterial?
(2)

- *S. pneumo*
- Non-typeable *H. flu*

(*M. catarrhalis* causes <10 % of all acute OM, with S. pyogenes still causing some cases)

Pain or fever continuing 3 days after antibiotic treatment has been started for acute otitis media = treatment failure. What about otorrhea or a bulging TM?

Otorrhea or bulging TM after 3 days are both treatment failures –
Switch meds!

Why is developing a cholesteatoma a problem?

1. It erodes & destroys the bones (ossicles, mastoid, etc.)
2. Often produces a nasty ear discharge

What *is* a cholesteatoma?

Keratinized squamous epithelium that
is not shed properly –
It forms a ball

How is a cholesteatoma usually
described on physical exam?

Pearly & superior,
at the margin of the TM

What are "screamer's nodules?"

Nodules that develop on the cords due
to overuse

What is the significance of screamer's
nodules?

Makes the voice hoarse

If you palpate a solid mass in the
sternocleidomastoid of an infant,
what is it likely to be?
(especially if the infant holds his or
her head in an odd position)

Torticollis

(contracted/spasmed muscle is the mass)

**If a neck mass is described as soft
and "spongy," it is likely to be what
diagnosis?**

Cystic hygroma

**If a patient has biphasic stridor &
a cutaneous hemangioma, what
should you consider as a possible
explanation?**

**Hemangioma at the glottis
(or subglottic)**

Must be eliminated due to airway risk!

**Can a foreign body produce
stridor?**

Yes

(If it is intrathoracic, it will be *expiratory*
stridor)

If you suspect that vascular
compression of the airway is causing
your patient's stridor (expiratory),
how do you evaluate that?

Barium swallow –
Shows *posterior* compression of the
esophagus

**Which type of vascular
compression of the airway will
barium swallow miss?**

Anterior compression –
**Usually due to an aberrant innominate
artery**

**How does unilateral choanal atresia
usually present?**

**Unilateral rhinorrhea in later infancy/
early childhood**

If a child begins to ignore things the caregiver asks her to do, and usually turns up the TV volume a little whenever she starts to watch TV, what should you suspect?

Conductive hearing loss

Is there anything you can do for a child with conductive hearing loss?

Yes –
Hearing aide, or sometimes surgical correction (depending on the cause)

Hearing loss that occurs after a significant head trauma or blast injury is usually due to what type of problem?

TM perforation & disruption of ossicles

Does otitis media with effusion cause a big decrease in hearing?

**Usually not –
It is mild & intermittent
(but still important)**

Do cholesteatomas usually cause hearing loss?

No, not by themselves
(If they open the TM or erode the ossicles, though, that will be a problem!)

What is tympanosclerosis?

Opacification & slight thickening of the TM

(usually develops in response to multiple bouts of OM)

What is the impact of tympanosclerosis on hearing?

Slight (conductive) hearing loss

Does having small or malformed ears impact a person's hearing (ears meaning the pinna or outer ear)?

**Yes –
But correction is easy via hearing aide or surgery**

Congenital syndromes that have sensorineural hearing loss as one of the problems mainly fall into two categories. What are they? (exclude in utero infections)

**1. Syndromes with cleft lip & palate
2. CHARGE syndrome**

How do you definitively test
for hearing problems in a child less
than 6 months old?

**BAER or ABR
(stands for: Brainstem Auditory
Evoked Response or
Auditory Brainstem Response)**

What does an auditory brainstem
response tell you?
(3)

- Whether there is hearing loss
- Whether it's conductive or
  sensorineural
- Whether one or both ears are affected

How can an auditory brainstem
response provide so much
information?

It follows the electrical path of CNS
processing from the moment the sound is
heard until it is completely processed

What is an appropriate screening test
for hearing in infants <6 months old,
since ABR is so complicated?

Behavioral Observational
Audiometry

**Which patient group should have
hearing tested with conventional,
pure tone audiometry?**

School-aged & older

**How specific is the information
provided by conventional pure tone
audiometry?**

**Specific –
Tests each ear separately &
discriminates sensorineural &
conductive loss**

When would you choose visual
reinforcement audiometry (VRA) to
evaluate for possible hearing loss?

Preschool kids –
Screens for *bilateral* hearing loss

**A child is being treated for a
perforated TM, but foul smelling
discharge persists. What diagnosis
was missed (or developed)?**

Cholesteatoma

Do some kids have congenital reasons
for persisting effusion after OM
infection?

Yes –
Some have floppy Eustachian tubes
or defective opening mechanisms

What nearby structure sometimes
causes or contributes to middle-ear
effusion?

Adenoid hypertrophy/tonsil hypertrophy

The sudden onset of bilateral sensorineural hearing loss can develop for a number of reasons. What is the infectious one?

Viral labyrinthitis

When sensorineural hearing loss occurs with a viral labyrinthitis, what is the prognosis for hearing?

It varies –
No treatment available, just wait & see

If sensorineural hearing loss develops due to medication toxicity, what will the patient complain of?

High-pitched tinnitus

If a child presents with sudden onset of unsteadiness & hearing loss, what diagnosis should you think of?

Perilymphatic fistula

What is a perilymphatic fistula?

A communication between the middle & inner ear (that allows the inner ear fluid to leak & be disrupted)

Aside from the obvious problems a perilymphatic fistula causes, what important complication do you have to watch out for?

Meningitis with otitis media infections

If "refer for specialty consultation" is an option in a perilymphatic fistula question, is it likely to be the right answer?

Yes –
Pediatric exams are not big on specialist consultations, but this is one diagnosis that needs it

How can you confirm a perilymphatic fistula diagnosis?

ENT has to do a tympanotomy & look

How is the presentation of a perilymphatic fistula different from Meniere disease?

Meniere adds tinnitus
(hearing loss, unsteadiness, & tinnitus)

How common is Meniere disease in children?

Very uncommon

If you are really motivated to identify the cause of rhinorrhea, what (unusual) lab procedure could you do?	Nasal smear
If rhinorrhea is due to seasonal allergies, what kind of cells do you expect to see on a smear?	Eos! (and a mix of other cells, of course)
If an adolescent has trouble with a chronic stuffy nose, what cause should you consider?	**Cocaine use**
When adolescents have a sinus infection, they present like adults. How do children with sinusitis present?	**Rhinorrhea** **Nasal congestion** **Cough** **Foul-smelling breath** **+/− Fever**
What are the typical sinusitis pathogens? (3)	Pneumococcus Non-typeable *H. flu* Moraxella catarrhalis
If a preschooler develops sinusitis, what is first-line treatment?	Amoxicillin
If sinusitis causes a cough, when is the cough especially noticeable?	**Nighttime**
If orbital cellulitis develops from a sinus infection, which sinus is most likely to be the culprit?	Ethmoid – Right beside the eyes & only separated by a very thin bone
If you are going to treat a patient for sinusitis, will the results of either a nasal or throat culture help you to determine the best antibiotic choice?	No – The results from nose & throat don't correlate well with results of sinus aspiration (the best way to get accurate data)
Why might you confuse strep pharyngitis with EBV on physical exam?	**Can cause thick exudate on tonsils** **&** **Palatal petechiae**
How long does the high fever phase of EBV last?	Often 1–2 weeks

Sore throat with exudate and hepatosplenomegaly is likely to be _____?

EBV

Should the liver be tender to palpation, if the patient has EBV?

Can be –
About 50 % are tender

If you have a patient with exudative pharyngitis, fever, & cervical lymphadenopathy, you may not be sure whether you're dealing with Strep or EBV. If you send a rapid strep & it's positive, what is it safe to conclude?

**Nothing –
Strep tests are sometimes falsely positive with EBV infection**

(or the patient could be a Strep carrier)

What differentiates EBV mononucleosis from Strep pharyngitis?

Longer duration
Hepatosplenomegaly

How long will the monospot test remain positive after a patient contracts mono?

Nine months

Definitive diagnosis of EBV acute mononucleosis is based on what criteria/criterion?

+ EBV Ig<u>M</u>

Progressive hoarseness that improves at adolescence, is better in the morning, and is not accompanied by any other findings or complaints is probably due to _____?

Vocal cord nodules

What is the treatment of choice for Strep pharyngitis?

Penicillin

(waiting for culture results will not change treatment outcome)

Some controversy now exists as to whether antibiotic treatment is appropriate, as the risk of serious antibiotic adverse effects is higher in some areas than the risk of developing rheumatic fever. Most practitioners still treat it, however.

If a patient develops a peritonsillar abscess, should the tonsil be removed?

Only if it recurs

What organism is most often found in peritonsillar abscesses?

β-Hemolytic strep

(anaerobes are also common)

If you ask a peritonsillar patient to "open wide" so you can see the pharynx, what is likely to happen?

They *don't* open wide – they have *trismus* (pain with opening the mouth)

Apparent torticollis, or a hyperextended neck, with enlargement of the retropharyngeal area on lateral neck X-ray in a child <4 years old is probably what diagnosis?

Retropharyngeal abscess

To differentiate it from epiglottitis, will retropharyngeal abscess kids drool, & will they sit up & forward?

Drool – sometimes

Sit up & forward – No
They usually lie down & may hyperextend or hold the neck in funny positions

If a patient sits "up and forward," how is that sometimes described in the medical literature?
  (single word)

Tripod
(or "tripod-ing")

Peritonsillar abscesses are most common in what age group?

Adolescents

Retropharyngeal abscesses usually occur in what age group?

<4 years old

Malformations of the external & middle ear should make you consider malformations of what other structure?

The kidney

(unless it is just ear tags)

If an infant develops cervical adenitis, what is it usually due to, and how is it managed?

- **Staph aureus**
- **IV antibiotics (such as clindamycin or vancomycin) are given – if inadequate response, then surgical drainage**

If a child has cervical adenitis due to atypical mycobacteria, will this affect the PPD?

Yes, but it will be <10 mm

If your patient has bacterial lymphadenopathy, what sort of antibiotics should you start with?

β-Lactamase-resistant antibiotics

(clindamycin, amoxicillin/clavulanate, cephalosporins, etc., depending on the local resistance patterns)

An unusual cause of croup that could only develop in children who have not had the usual immunizations is _____?

**Measles
(rubeola)**

What is the most common "tumor" of the larynx in children?

**Papillomas
(kind of a tumor)**

How are laryngeal papillomas treated?

Excision
(via laser)

Do laryngeal papillomas have a potential for malignant transformation?

Yes – not often, though

Why do spasmodic croup patients not usually seem ill?

**It is thought to be an allergy problem
(more common in atopics)**

What are the other names for bacterial tracheitis?

**Pseudomembranous croup
(presents like croup, but has thicker secretions)
Or
Membranous laryngotracheitis
Or
Laryngotracheobronchitis**

What position will a bacterial tracheitis patient usually be found in?

Supine
(They're sick – they want to lie down + it helps to drain the secretions)

A sick patient with inspiratory stridor, a barking cough, and thick nasty sputum is likely to have what diagnosis?

Bacterial tracheitis

You are examining a patient, and see 4–5 mm ulcers on the posterior pharynx. She has had a fever for several days, and is reluctant to eat. What is the likely diagnosis?

Herpangina/
Coxsackie virus

The oral lesions of Coxsackie virus are often accompanied by lesions on what other part(s) of the body?

Hands & feet –
As in "hand, foot, & mouth disease"

When Coxsackie virus causes herpangina, will lesions of the hands & feet also appear?

Often, but not always

When Coxsackie virus does cause hand or foot lesions, what will the lesions look like?

Vesiculopapular

What is the typical presentation of a herpes simplex "cold sore?"

**Painful vesicles –
Often at the vermillion border of the lip**

(First episode accompanied by fever & adenopathy)

Some people get ulcers in the mouth that come & go, and are painful. They often develop following minor trauma to the area, but the cause is not really clear. What are these ulcers called?

Aphthous ulcers

What does an aphthous ulcer look like?
(3 aspects)

Gray-white ulcer
Thin rim of bright red
Usually on mucosa (not gingiva)

If a patient develops periorbital swelling due to a dental problem, what is the likely problem?

Maxillary dental abscess

If a patient develops swelling under the jaw due to a dental problem, what is the likely cause?

Mandibular tooth abscess

Delayed eruption of tooth is associated with which endocrine problems?

Hypothyroidism
&
Hypopituitarism

What disordered development leads   Ectodermal hypoplasia
to delayed tooth eruption?

Name the nutritional syndrome that   Rickets
causes delayed tooth eruption?

Decreased ability to sweat –   Delayed tooth eruption
hypohidrosis – is associated with what
dental problem?

If a patient has a bifid uvula, what oral   Cleft palate hidden under the soft tissue
abnormality is often found?
                                             (aka "submucous" cleft palate)

**Midline, anterior, neck cysts   Thyroglossal
are often what specific sort of cyst?**

**Is it a good idea to remove   Usually not –
thyroglossal cysts?   May contain the only functional
                                           thyroid tissue**

**If an infant has tender red nodules,   Cold exposure –
and "deep-seated" plaques on the   Diagnosis is "cold-induced
cheek, but seems to be otherwise   panniculitis"**
well, what environmental cause
could be the problem?**   (usually via a cold water-filled pacifier,
                                           or something similar)

What is the treatment for cold-induced   Nothing –
panniculitis?   Observe & it will resolve in a week or so

If a child is diagnosed with   "Go to OR to evaluate under anesthesia"
epiglottitis, what is the correct
disposition from the ED/office?

If a child has recurrent OM infections,   • Submucosal (hidden) cleft palate
and a bifid uvula, what is the likely   • Bilateral myringotomy tubes are often
problem & solution?   needed

Chapter 11
General Adolescent Medicine and Relevant Gynecology Question and Answer Items

Roughly speaking, what is the definition of an "adolescent?"	10–21 years old
In the USA, what is the most common reason for 15–24-year-olds to visit a general outpatient clinic, if they are female?	**Pregnancy!**
Adolescents are frequent visitors to emergency departments. What are male adolescents usually seen for?	**Injuries (usually non-urgent)**
What complaints most often bring adolescent girls to the emergency department? (3 categories)	Sore throat, abdominal pain, & pregnancy/sexual activity-related conditions
What is the leading cause of death for African-American adolescents?	**Homicide**
What is the leading cause of adolescent death & injury, for all adolescents together?	**Car & motorcycle collisions**
Risky behaviors during adolescence lead to this common cause of morbidity & mortality for Hispanic and African-American 24–44-year-olds. What is it?	HIV

© Springer Science+Business Media New York 2016
C.M. Houser, *Pediatric Tricky Topics, Volume 2*,
DOI 10.1007/978-1-4939-3109-5_11

What is the typical age for onset of puberty in African-American girls, and what is the range?	• **8 years** • **Range is 6–10 years**
How long does puberty usually last for girls?	**4 years**
How long does puberty usually last for boys?	**3 years**
What is the typical age for onset of puberty for Caucasian girls? (average & range)	• **About 10 years** • **Range is 8–11 ½ years**
When do boys typically begin puberty? (average & range)	• **11 ½ years** • **Range 9 ½–13 ½**
In relation to Tanner stage, when do girls usually have their adolescent growth spurt?	**Tanner stage 2 or 3**
When do boys usually have their growth spurt, in relation to Tanner stage?	**Later –** **Tanner 4**
About what proportion of total skeletal height growth occurs during adolescence?	¼ (some sources indicate as much as ½)
What is the male pattern for lean body mass and fat percentage changes during adolescence?	• ↑ lean body mass • Small early ↑ in body fat (about 10 %)
Does respiratory rate increase or decrease during adolescence?	Decreases (Remember, it's heading toward the adult value)
Both boys & girls have a change in normal pulmonary function during adolescence. In particular, for the FEV_1/FVC ratio, what happens?	It decreases (The ratio falls during childhood, then increases somewhat during the growth spurt of adolescence)

What impressive change occurs in the size of the heart in adolescent boys?

It doubles!!

What is the average age for menarche?

12 ¾ years
(the average for African-American girls is somewhat younger)

What is usually the first sign of sexual maturation in a girl?

Thelarche
(development of breast buds)

In terms of sexual maturation, are boys more likely to have a *negative* self-image if they develop early or late?

Late

In terms of sexual maturation, are girls more likely to have a *positive* self-image if they develop early or late?

Late is more positive

(so it's opposite in girls vs. boys)

In early adolescence (ages 10–13), most kids have difficulty with what type of behavioral regulation?

Impulse control
(and they usually also lack insight/ability to think about impulse control)

On the boards, if a health issue needs to be discussed with a 10–13-year-old, what are the "buzzwords" for how you should do that?
(3)

- **Simple, clear language**
- **Direct communication**
- **Visual & verbal "cues" should be used**

Who has their adolescent growth spurt earlier – girls or boys?

Girls do!

(Don't they always say that "girls develop earlier?")

Middle adolescents (14–16 years) have completed or nearly completed puberty. What is the most important force in their lives for support and change?

Peers

At what point in adolescence do individual relationships become more important than the peer group, as a whole?

Late adolescence
(17–21 years)

What are the top three reasons adolescents are hospitalized, in general terms?

1. Pregnancy
2. Psychiatric disorders
3. Injuries

Although specific guidelines vary from state to state, emancipated minors are generally defined as . . .? (4 criteria)	1. **In the military** 2. **Married** 3. **Has children** 4. **Living independently & financially self-supporting**
If you are required to notify parents of a minor child's treatment, what must you do first?	**Inform the minor**
Is parental consent required for emergency treatment of a minor?	No – No consent is needed
What situations always require the physician to break confidentiality?	1. **Child abuse/elder abuse** 2. **Danger to self or others**
Should adolescents be seen alone or with the parent(s)?	**Alone (at least for part of the time)**
What is the guiding principle in providing adolescent health care?	**Autonomy – Give them as much autonomy as they wish, unless legal or safety concerns prevent it**
What special areas are important to ask about in adolescent exams? (4 about the individual & 2 about relationships)	1. Peer & family relationships 2. Depression 3. Sexual relationships/activity 4. Substance use 5. Eating disorders 6. Self-image and school
What psychiatric problems are especially big issues in adolescents?	Depression & Eating disorders
If you are legally required to report treatment of a minor, when the minor does not wish you to inform his or her parents, what are you supposed to recommend?	**Bring the parents into the discussion, with the pediatrician as "facilitator" for the discussion**

What self-exam techniques should you instruct adolescents about?

Girls – breast self-awareness (breast self-exam per se is no longer mandatory, but it is an acceptable option)

Boys – testicular exam (no proven benefit, however)

What sensory screening exams are important for adolescents, and why?

Vision – myopia sometimes occurs with the growth spurt

Hearing – due to the loud music

When should young women have their first pelvic exam? (3 situations)

1. Vaginal discharge
2. Complaint of menstrual problems or pelvic pain
3. Reaches age 21

(Note: This is a change – previous recommendations were to institute pelvic exams between ages 11 & 21, depending on history/risk factors)

What two important cardiovascular risk factors should be screened for in adolescents?

Hypertension & dyslipidemia

(Note: Dyslipidemia screening is a recent addition! The dyslipidemia screen is recommended early, between ages 9 & 11 years)

What orthopedic issue should be screened for in adolescents?

Scoliosis

(>10 % curvature *requires* ortho referral)

How often should adolescents have routine exams, if they have no complaints?

Yearly (for preventative care)

Should sexually active adolescents be routinely screened for STDs?

Yes – & risk assessment for STDs should be conducted each year

Should HIV screening be routinely conducted with adolescent patients?

Yes – Between ages 16 & 18

Should the routine genital exam of an adolescent girl include a Pap smear?

No – Routine internal examination with or without a speculum is no longer recommended

Which psychiatric disorder should be routinely screened for in adolescent patients?

Depression –
screen yearly, due to risk of suicide in this group (along with other depression-related morbidity)

What immunizations are *usually* given in adolescence?
  (6 in total)

- **Tdap booster (around age 11 years)**
- **Meningococcus & HPV (beginning around age 11 years)**
- **Annual influenza vaccinations**
- **MMR & Varicella (this is the second dose – they are given in early adolescence if the second dose was not given during early childhood)**

If a child has chronic liver disease, what extra immunization should you give (in addition to the routine ones)?

Hepatitis A

What is the recommended standard of care for how often you should provide routine health guidance to an adolescent's care giver(s)?

Yearly

At the yearly visit, what sorts of health guidance should you provide to an adolescent?
  (4 categories)

1. Injury prevention (especially seat belt & helmet use, weapons safety, violence avoidance, & importance of exercise)
2. Diet info
3. Sexual behavior info
4. Substance abuse info

Especially for sports-oriented adolescent boys, what substance abuse topic needs to be addressed?

Anabolic steroids

If a child engages in one type of risky behavior, is he or she more or less likely to engage in others?

MORE

Which gender is more likely to smoke – girls or boys?

Girls

Which gender is more likely to drink alcohol?	**Boys** **(by a lot!)**
How common is marijuana use in adolescents?	At least 50 %
What is the average of first use for marijuana?	14 years
What are the biggest behavioral markers of kids who are at risk for substance abuse?	**Poor impulse control/"unnecessary" aggressive outbursts**
Which psychiatric disorders put adolescents at special risk for substance abuse?	**Depression & anxiety disorders**
What are the main factors in the child's environment that put the adolescent at risk for substance abuse? **(2)**	1. **Peer group use** 2. **Household drug use** **(especially by parents)**
What social changes in an adolescent's life are warning signs for possible substance abuse?	• **Increasing emotional/physical isolation** • **New peer group members**
What warning signs for possible substance abuse can be noted at school? **(3)**	• **Decrease in school performance** • **Increased absences** • **Decreased interest in sports or other school activities**
If an adolescent is involved in a crime, should this make you worry that substance abuse could be an issue?	**Yes**
What learning difference <u>greatly</u> increases the probability that an adolescent will get involved in substance abuse?	**ADD or ADHD** **(Attention-deficit disorder or attention-deficit hyperactivity disorder)**

What is the "mature minor" rule for provision of health care?

Low risk care that is clearly of benefit to the minor can be provided if the minor understands the risks & benefits

Is it all right to perform a urine drug screening without an adolescent's permission?

Generally, no

Which fairly common psychedelic recreational drug is not identified by most urine toxicology screens?

LSD

Before puberty, depression is equally common in boys & girls.
In adolescence, which group is more often clinically depressed?

Girls
(2–3× more)

What unusual presentation does depression in an adolescent sometimes have?

Boredom

The main manifestation of clinical depression is depressed mood or irritability with loss of interest in things. Adolescents are also likely to have what weight & appetite changes?

(3)

1. **Weight loss _or gain_**
2. **Appetite decrease _or increase_**
3. **Failure of weight to increase appropriately to overall size**

How long should symptoms of depression be present to allow a diagnosis of "major depressive disorder?"

More than 2 weeks
(without an identifiable stressor)

What cognitive and specific emotional changes are markers of depression in adolescents?

(4)

1. **Difficulty thinking/ concentrating**
2. **Recurrent thoughts of death**
3. **Guilt**
4. **Worthlessness**

To make the diagnosis of major depressive disorder, the general requirement of depressed or irritable mood with diminished interest must be met, plus what else?	**4 out of 9 associated symptoms (weight issues, cognitive & specific emotional items, sleep, energy, & psychomotor changes)**
The associated sleep disturbance accompanying depression in adolescents is _____ ?	**Either insomnia *or* too much sleep**
In terms of psychomotor activity level, what is expected with depression in adolescents?	**Can either increase *or* decrease**
For the associated depression symptom that has to do with fatigue/energy level, what is expected?	**Low energy/increased fatigue**
Do the boards like asking about depression in adolescents?	**Yes!**
If symptoms of depression are present, but an identifiable stressor *has occurred* in the past 3 months, what is the correct diagnosis?	**Adjustment disorder with depressed mood (Note: Adjustment disorders are considered to be "stress-response syndromes" in the new DSM V)**
When depression or another major psychiatric disorder is suspected in an adolescent, what other types of problems should you consider? (4)	1. Substance abuse 2. Chronic systemic illness (like SLE) 3. Thyroid disease 4. Nutritional issues
How does the age of onset for depression affect the expected course of the disorder?	Earlier onset = more severe disease & more recurrences
How long will major depression usually last if it is not treated?	About 8 months

When is it all right to hospitalize an adolescent for psychiatric reasons? **(4)**	**The usual –** 1. **Danger to self or others** 2. **Not responding to outpatient treatment** 3. **Mania** 4. **Treatment is complicated by active substance abuse**
What are the typical meds used for bipolar disorder?	1. **Valproic acid (for mania) & lamotrigine (for depression)** 2. **Carbamazepine (for both)** 3. **Lithium (for both – tox issues are a problem with adolescents, especially)** **(antipsychotic agents are also helpful in some patients)**
How is bipolar disorder different from regular depression?	**There is cycling in the mood (length of cycle varies), and many patients experience mania as well as depression** *Mania is not absolutely necessary, though*
What is the other name for a cycling mood disorder?	Cyclothymic disorder (cyclo = cycling) (thymic = emotion)
What is dysthymic disorder? (dys = bad) (thymic = mood)	Chronic depressed mood for at least 1 year that doesn't meet criteria for major depression
Are multiple psychiatric disorders often present in the same individual?	Yes
What is the preferred pharmaceutical treatment for depression in adolescents?	**SSRIs** **(serotonin reuptake inhibitors)**
Why are SSRIs preferred to TCAs (tricyclic antidepressants) for medication-based treatment of depression?	1. **More effective in this population** 2. **Much safer**

Eating disorders are more common in which gender?

Girls

(10:1)

How common is anorexia nervosa among girls (in %)?

About 1 % of girls

(sources vary – lifetime prevalence 0.3–4 %)

What is the most common age of onset for anorexia nervosa?

13–18 years

(research suggests about 85 % have onset during this age range)

Is it common for anorexia to develop in very young adolescent girls, <13 years old?

It is less common than in the older teens, but still occurs regularly

(data on how common it is are quite mixed)

Girls who participate in what three athletic activities are notorious for having higher rates of eating disorders?

(very popular test item)

Gymnastics, ballet, figure skating

What personality traits are often present in the girls who later develop anorexia?

Perfectionism/overachievers

Do anorectics usually announce that they are going on a diet, when they first begin to manifest the disorder?

Yes

What is often occurring in the adolescent's life, when anorexia first appears?

Transition or stressful events (e.g., beginning at a new school level)

Data is quite mixed as to whether negative events are actually related to the onset of adolescent eating disorders or not

Anorexia has what effect on the sex hormones secreted by both boys & girls affected by the disorder?

Suppresses them

There were four diagnostic criteria for anorexia. Which one has been eliminated in DSM V?

No menstrual criteria
(Absence of three *consecutive* cycles was previously a criterion)

One of the criteria for anorexia has to do with an unusual fear. What is it?

<u>Intense</u> **fear of becoming obese, which *doesn't decrease as weight loss occurs***

What is strange about the body image of adolescents with anorexia?

They "see" themselves as fat, even if they are abnormally thin

(altered body image)

What is the behavioral criterion in the diagnostic criteria for anorexia nervosa?

<u>Inability</u> **to maintain a minimally normal body weight**

(the term "refusal" has been eliminated, because it implied a conscious intent not to maintain body weight, which is not necessarily the case)

In addition to calorie restriction & excessive exercise, what other behaviors do anorectics sometimes engage in, which are especially likely to cause serious problems?
(3)

1. Vomiting
2. Diuretic use
3. Laxative abuse

What electrolyte disturbances are especially common in anorexia?

Hypokalemia

&

Hypochloremic metabolic alkalosis (due to vomiting)

Why might anorectics be anemic, aside from nutritional issues?

Anorexia tends to suppress the bone marrow – both RBCs and WBCs may be low

In general, anorexia nervosa is associated with a lowering of many body functions & secretions. What is elevated in anorectics?

Cortisol

&

Endorphins

Due to the very low amount of body fat, anorectics are at especially high risk for what environmental problem?

Hypothermia

What is the most life-threatening aspect of anorexia nervosa?

Cardiac arrhythmias due to electrolyte derangements

(not starvation – although that is also possible)

What is the best way to evaluate an anorectic for risk of serious cardiac arrhythmias?

Exercise stress testing –

Prolonged QT or ST depression during exercise stress testing = high risk

What is a common, but less life-threatening, cardiac rhythm problem often seen in anorectics?

Bradycardia

Severe anorectics are at risk for CHF (congestive heart failure) if what treatment is initiated too rapidly?

Hydration

When treatment for anorexia is initiated, is it all right for weight gain to occur as rapidly as possible?

Slow gain is best to decrease complications

(About 1/3 kg per day is the maximum)

Which is more common, bulimia or anorexia?

Bulimia

What is the typical weight for a bulimic patient – normal, overweight, or underweight?

Normal or slightly overweight

Is it possible to have both anorexia & bulimia?

Yes –
Or some patients alternate between the two

At what age does bulimia typically begin?

Mid-to-late adolescence

In addition to metabolic alkalosis & hypokalemia, what other lab value might be abnormal in a bulimic patient?

Amylase (elevated)

Lots of people get sore throats. Why do bulimics have sore throats?

Vomiting

Are bulimics at risk for cardiac arrhythmia?

Yes –
It just depends how far out of whack they get their electrolytes

What special & rather unusual findings are you supposed to look for when bulimia is suspected (especially on the boards)?

(3)

(very popular test item)

1. Missing tooth enamel (on the inner surface – due to stomach acid with vomiting)
2. Bilaterally swollen parotid glands
3. Calluses on the dorsum of the fingers (from inducing vomiting)

What other psychiatric disorders are often coexistent with bulimia?

(2 groups)

Affective disorders
Obsessive-compulsive disorder(s)

What characteristic eating pattern is seen in bulimia?

Binging & purging

What are the three easiest-to-remember criteria for bulimia?

1. Binge eating (multiple times – not just once)
2. Feeling "out of control"
3. Purging/dieting/exercising

In order to differentiate bulimics from folks eating Thanksgiving dinner, what other bingeing criteria was added?

Average of ≥1 binge/week *for at least 3 months*

(the same frequency criterion is used for "binge eating disorder," which features mainly the food binging behavior, without the other aspects of bulimia nervosa)

There are a total of five diagnostic criteria for bulimia. What are they?

1. Binge eating
2. Feeling out of control about bingeing
3. Inappropriate compensatory behavior (purging/dieting/exercise/ laxatives)
4. Persistent binging (avg of ≥1 time/ week × 3 months)
5. Ongoing concern about body shape or weight

What medication group is often helpful in bulimia, and sometimes helpful in anorexia?	SSRIs
Is pharmacotherapy alone usually successful with either bulimia or anorexia nervosa?	**No –** **Therapy, behavior modification, & nutritional guidance are usually also needed**
Is asymmetric breast growth in an adolescent reason for alarm?	**No –** **It is common & may be present even in adulthood**
What is the most common breast mass in an adolescent?	**A fibroadenoma**
The initial breast development, the breast bud, is made up of what types of tissues? (3)	1. Ductal tissue 2. Stromal tissue 3. Fat
Later breast development, after the breast bud, is mainly comprised of growth in what two histological parts of the breast?	1. Ductal 2. "Lobular-alveolar"
Fibrocystic changes are most often symptomatic in what part of the breast?	Upper outer quadrant
The hallmark of fibrocystic breast cysts is _____?	Cyclic changes with the menstrual cycle
How common is accessory breast tissue or more than the usual two nipples?	Common – 1–2 % of females
Where will polymastia (accessory breast tissue) and extra nipples be found?	Along the mammalian "breast line" (running vertically down the chest, like on a cat or dog)
What is the special word for more than two nipples?	Polythelia
How is the discomfort of fibrocystic breast tissue managed? (3 strategies)	1. NSAIDs 2. Breast support (a good bra) 3. Oral contraceptives

Is mammography a good way to evaluate a breast mass in an adolescent?

No –
The tissue is too dense

When should an otherwise not concerning breast mass be evaluated further in an adolescent girl?

If it lasts more than 3 cycles

(at the same size or larger)

How should a breast mass be evaluated initially, after physical exam?

Needle aspiration

If needle aspiration of a breast mass does not provide a definitive answer about the type of mass, what should be done?

Excisional biopsy

Nonpregnant adolescents sometimes develop mastitis. How should you treat it in this group?
   (3 strategies)

1. Antibiotics (PO)
2. Pain management
3. Local heat application

Which organism is the most likely cause of mastitis in an adolescent?

Staph aureus

Mastitis is most common in what two groups?

Newborns

&

Lactating women

A painless, rubbery, breast mass that does not change with hormonal variation is probably a _____?

Fibroadenoma

(no malignancy issues – usually found in the upper outer quadrant)

What is the *most common* cause of secondary amenorrhea?

Pregnancy

Amenorrhea + difficulty smelling (anosmia) =

Kallman's syndrome

What is the most common pituitary cause of amenorrhea?

Prolactin-secreting tumor (usually prolactinoma)

If a pituitary tumor is causing amenorrhea, what other symptom is often present, especially on the boards?

Galactorrhea

Cystosarcoma phyllodes tumors sometimes occur in pediatric patients. Is the cystosarcoma phyllodes breast tumor malignant?

No, but it can become malignant

What is one important hallmark of a cystosarcoma phyllodes tumor?

Rapid growth

Although breast cancer is very rare in adolescents, how does it present?
(3)

- Hard, fixed mass
- Nipple involvement
- Overlying skin changes

What findings automatically mean that a breast mass requires biopsy?
(3)

1. **Bloody nipple discharge**
2. **Nipple retraction or other involvement**
3. **Skin dimpling or other overlying changes**

What proportion of teenage girls has dysmenorrhea?

>2/3

What causes dysmenorrhea?

Prostaglandin increases → uterine muscle contractions and vasoconstriction

Why is dysmenorrhea an important issue for adolescents, aside from discomfort?

It is a big cause of school absenteeism

On the topics of sex and substance use/abuse, should you maintain an adolescent's confidentiality or involve parents?

Maintain confidentiality *unless* the adolescent requests or consents to parental involvement

Why are follow-up visits especially important for adolescents?

They sometimes need two visits to disclose what's really bothering them

(The chief complaint is often not the real complaint.)

If a dipstick UA is positive in a sexually active male adolescent, what should you consider, in addition to a possible UTI?

Leukocytes in the urine can alert you to an asymptomatic STD

(Real screening for GC & chlamydia is even better, of course)

Which adolescents should definitely be screened for cholesterol?

Everyone between ages 9 & 11

+

More frequent monitoring for those with a family history of:
Hyperlipidemia
Early cardiovascular disease
Comorbidities such as obesity, diabetes, or
hypertension

Are patients and family members reliable historians about whether your patient has had varicella?

Positive history is usually reliable

Negative history not very reliable

If a question indicates that there is no "reliable history" of chicken pox, what should you do about immunizing the adolescent?

Immunize or check titers then decide

(previous chicken pox is not a contraindication to giving the vaccine, so it is sometimes more time & resource effective to give it than to titer first)

If a younger patient's previous history of varicella is unclear, what options are acceptable with regard to varicella immunization?

Immunize anyway

Or

Check titers & immunize if it is low or absent

What is the most effective way, in general, to help adolescents develop good behaviors?

Model them
(including having some adolescents model the behaviors for other adolescents)

What special safety issues should you address with parents of adolescents?

1. Securing dangerous or "entertaining" medications
2. Security of household weapons
3. Monitoring & managing new drivers

How many Tanner stages are there?

Five

Is there a Tanner stage zero?

No!

Is it helpful to tell adolescents about healthful behaviors (seat belt use, good diet, etc.)?

Yes –
Even if they don't seem to be listening

On the boards, if you're looking for the right answer, and the question involves a female, what should you look for?

"Pregnancy" or "pregnancy test" is often right!!!

When interviewing an adolescent, should you wait for them to bring up sensitive topics, or be proactive about it?

Proactive –
When the doctor brings up the topic, it often helps them to discuss their concerns

Which group of males is at unusually high risk for eating disorders?

Wrestlers & rowers

(overfocus on weight due to importance of being as light as possible to qualify for a more advantageous weight class – & some tradition of attempting to dehydrate or purge to lose weight acutely before sporting events)

It is even more difficult to make a psychiatric diagnosis in an adolescent than it usually would be, because their moods & behavior are often "difficult." What clue will the boards usually give you to indicate a psychiatric/substance abuse problem?

A "change" in the pattern of behavior or peer group

How common is gynecomastia in adolescent boys?

Very common
(about 50 %)

What are the usual physical findings in male gynecomastia?
(3)

Usually but often asymmetric enlargement

<4 cm

+/– tenderness

If an adolescent has a bout of clinical depression, how likely is he or she to suffer another bout over the next 5 years?

About 45 % will have another episode in 5 years

If an adolescent appears in a vignette with what seems to be mastitis, <u>but</u> she is not pregnant and the discharge is bloody, what should you consider?

Breast cancer!

Bloody discharge =
Breast cancer until proven otherwise

If mastitis is presented in a non-pregnant female, what should you consider?

Breast cancer

(infectious mastitis is possible, *but unlikely*, without pregnancy)

What is the most common cause of secondary amenorrhea?

Pregnancy

Can pregnancy cause primary amenorrhea?

Yes –
If pregnancy occurs at just the right time

What is anatomic amenorrhea?

When mechanical problems in the anatomy prevent menstruation

How does anatomic amenorrhea present?

With pain –
The girl is menstruating, but it can't escape!

Which is more common – anatomic amenorrhea, or amenorrhea due to endocrine axis problems?

Endocrine axis problems
(hypothalamic – pituitary – ovarian – axis)

If a female adolescent presents with hirsutism & virilization, most of us think of PCOS. What else should you consider?
(3)

- **Anabolic steroid use**
- **Adrenal adenoma**
- **Cushing's syndrome**

What two evaluations *must* you always conduct if the chief complaint is amenorrhea, and why?

1. **Pregnancy test**
2. **Genital & consider pelvic exam –**
   otherwise you *can't* find an anatomic abnormality!

Epididymitis in an adolescent is usually due to which general group of organisms?

Sexually transmitted disease organisms

Any time an adolescent presents for an STD or pregnancy-related complaint, what should you also do?

HIV counseling!!!

Is breast asymmetry in female adolescents common?

Yes –
25 % will persist into adulthood

What is "juvenile hypertrophy" of a breast?

Massive enlargement of one or both breasts

What can you do for juvenile hypertrophy of the breasts?

Mammoplasty or hormonal treatment (progesterone or antiestrogens)

But for mammoplasty you have to wait until they've finished growing

If a breast mass in an adolescent is determined to be cystic (meaning it's a cyst), what should you do about it?

Observe

How common is it for an adolescent girl to have a breast mass?

Very common

How common is it for an adolescent girl to have breast cancer?

Vanishingly rare

When would "excisional biopsy" be the right answer for how to proceed with evaluation of a cystic mass in an adolescent breast?

Only if it's been aspirated

&

you got *bloody aspirate*

Why is mammography not helpful in adolescents?

The breast tissue is too dense

(not enough fat in it yet)

Although there are other things to think about, androgenization in an adolescent female should always make you consider what syndrome?

Polycystic ovary syndrome (PCOS)

What types of dysfunctional uterine bleeding are often seen in the pediatric population?	• **Anovulatory – has to do with hormonal regulation of menses** • **Ovulatory – a structural or bleeding disorder is causing the problem**
Dysfunctional uterine bleeding (DUB) is usually due to what cycling issue in adolescent patients?	**Anovulatory cycles** **(These are especially common in the 2 years following menarche)**
Hormonally speaking, what happens in most adolescent anovulatory cycles?	• **Lack of progesterone** • **Estrogen level is maintained (unopposed estrogen leads to increased endometrial lining build-up)**
If there is an unusual amount of bleeding at menarche, what should this make you consider?	**Bleeding disorder/diathesis**
What hematologic issues would be high on your list to investigate if there were an unusual amount of bleeding at menarche? **(top 4 possibilities)**	• **von Willebrand disease** • **Platelet dysfunction** • **Factor 8 or 9 deficiency** • **Thrombocytopenia**
An unusual amount of bleeding at menarche would be an unusual presentation of what fairly common disease of the blood?	Leukemia
One reason a pelvic exam should be performed on DUB patients is to identify what group of DUB causes?	Traumatic (lacerations, tears, foreign bodies)
Although dysmenorrhea is common in adolescents, there are three important causes of *secondary* dysmenorrhea you should consider. What are they?	1. *Ectopic (can be deadly)* 2. **Infection (including endometritis & PID)** 3. **Endometriosis**
What is the course of normal pubertal gynecomastia (<4 cm)?	**Spontaneous resolution**

When does the first discussion about contraception usually happen for an adolescent, relative to when they begin having sex?

Six months *after* they start having sex (or at a visit for a missed period)

Which cancer is seen in the female children of mothers who took DES (diethylstilbestrol)?

"Clear cell" adenocarcinoma –

Presents as DUB because it is an endometrial cancer

During what years was DES mainly used by pregnant mothers in the USA?

1940s through early 1970s –

(Use continued after that in some other countries, and it was not banned in the USA, just less popular)

Which form of contraception also prevents certain STDs?

Condoms

(male condoms, that is – female condoms provide more limited STD protection than the male version)

How effective are condoms at preventing pregnancy in real-world situations?

About 90 %

How effective are "female condoms" lat preventing pregnancy in real-world settings?

About 80 %

If a patient has a history of clotting problems (too much clotting) or strokes, can she still be a candidate for oral contraceptives?

No!

(Absolute contraindication)

If a patient has DUB, and the cause has not yet been determined, is she a candidate for oral contraceptives?

No!

(Absolute contraindication – could be promoting a hormone dependent cancer, etc.)

If a patient has known liver disease, can oral contraceptives still be considered?

No!

(Absolute contraindication)

Which contraceptives are 100 %, or nearly 100 %, effective?

- **Abstinence**
- **IUDs & oral contraceptives are about 99 % with correct use**
- **Depo-Provera 99 %**

How effective is the "rhythm method" in preventing pregnancy in real-world settings?

About 80 % if used correctly

How effective is a diaphragm with spermicide in actual use?

80 %

(About the same as rhythm!)

A 13-year-old girl presents at menarche, with copious bleeding that drops her hematocrit to 21. The bleeding is difficult to control. What general category of problem should you consider?

Bleeding disorder

If a patient has a known estrogen-dependent tumor, should you avoid oral contraceptives?

You bet!

(Yes, definitely)

What is the other name for mifepristone?

RU-486

How effective is mifepristone at preventing pregnancy after unprotected intercourse?

100 % if taken within 72 h

What is the "morning after" pill?

An oral contraceptive regimen designed to decrease pregnancies after unprotected sex

What is the regimen for the "morning after" pill?

Patient takes 2–5 oral contraceptive pills in the first dose –
Same dose 12 h later

(the specific number of pills depends on the composition of the pills used)

What must the morning after pills contain to be effective, when combined oral contraceptives are used?

A *total* of about 100 µg *ethinylestradiol*

+

0.5–1.0 mg *levonorgestrel*

("Plan B" is two 0.75 mg tablets of levonorgestrel taken at one time)

When must counseling be provided with HIV testing?

Both before & after testing – every time!

How do you test for HIV?

- Initial screen is the ELISA
- Follow-up on a positive result with the Western blot to confirm it

Mnemonic:
Think of a nice lady named "Elisa," who is the secretary to a big executive. She "screens" the executive's calls.

An adolescent who is sexually active presents with fever, malaise, lymphadenopathy, and skin rash. What should be on your differential – especially for the boards?

(popular boards topic)

HIV! –
This is "acute retroviral syndrome" or acute seroconversion illness

When does the acute retroviral syndrome develop, relative to exposure to HIV?

Within a few weeks

If you are trying to evaluate for HIV infection in an adolescent who may have acute retroviral syndrome, what tests can you send?
(2)

PCR for:

HIV DNA

  Or

HIV plasma RNA

If you suspect acute retroviral syndrome, what tests for HIV are not useful?

- **ELISA**
- **Western blot**
- **Fluorescent antibodies (there is no significant antibody titer, yet)**

Is it important to know about HIV infection as early as the period when the patient has acute retroviral syndrome?

Yes –
Early treatment may be helpful

Although we try to keep care of sexually transmitted diseases confidential for adolescents, what breach of confidentiality is sometimes required by public health legislation?

Reporting of STDs

(the information is protected, though – even from subpoena in most states)

Which STDs are required to be reported, in all US states?

GC
Chlamydia
Syphilis
AIDS

(all of the classic ones + AIDS)

Hepatitis A vaccination is recommended for what three groups of adolescents?

1. Drug users (any type)
2. Men who have sex with men
3. Those who live or travel in endemic areas

What percentage of US teens has had sex by age 19?

71 %

(33 % by age 16 years)
(48 % by age 17 years)
(61 % by age 18 years)

Which group of adolescents has the highest rate of GC and chlamydia? (gender & age group)

Females aged 15–19 years

For female adolescents, what proportion have identifiable HPV DNA (human papillomavirus), if they are sexually active?

Estimated between 1/3 & 2/3

(To keep it simple, figure ½)

Which STI is most common in sexually active adolescents?

HPV
(still, despite availability of the vaccine)

Vaccination for HPV should reduce the percentage of adolescents carrying HPV DNA. Which patients are eligible for vaccination?

- Essentially all pediatric patients (male & female) are now considered eligible
- 11 years or older (Most effective prior to beginning sexual activity, *but may still be given after – this is a change!*)

What percentage of sexually active females age 14–19 years is infected with Chlamydia?

About 7 %
(2012 data)

(many are asymptomatic)

Although adolescents comprise only 25 % of the sexually active population, what percentage of STIs is found in this group?

50 %

(HPV, then chlamydia, & trichomonas are especially common)

If a pregnant adolescent is concerned about her options for delivery because she has HPV, what should you tell her?

Even if lesions are present at delivery, it is okay to deliver vaginally

This is a change – some used to recommend c-section

Under what circumstances would a pregnant patient with HPV be advised that she should not deliver vaginally?

If the lesions are very large, making delivery mechanically difficult

If a pregnant patient is known to have herpes, should you do serial cultures, to monitor for viral shedding?

No –
It's been studied & it's not useful

If a pregnant adolescent is known to have herpes, does this affect her delivery options?

Not unless lesions are present at the time of delivery

(A speculum exam should be done to check for intravaginal lesions before delivery – the mechanism of transmission to neonates, though, is not really clear)

If a pregnant adolescent is known to have herpes, what should you consider in the last trimester?

Suppressive therapy

(e.g., valacyclovir, acyclovir)

When is a herpes simplex infection likely to cause a big problem for the neonate?

If the *initial infection* occurs around the time of delivery

(fetal infection rates are quite high)

All pregnant adolescents should be offered what test?

(important boards topic!)

HIV

What percentage of adolescents has had sex by age 16, in the US?

33 %

Are adolescents able to consent to STI treatment independently, without a parent or caregiver's consent?

Yes, in all 50 US states

(some states do have minimum age requirements, however, usually of 14 years or less)

Although you are a pediatrician, what things are you supposed to know to do at the first prenatal visit?
(5)

1. **STD screen –**
   offers HIV testing
   does syphilis screening
   does Gonorrhea & Chlamydia cultures
2. **Heptitis screening – HepBsAg (Hepatitis B surface antigen)**
3. **Pap smear (if she hasn't had one in the past year)**
4. **Urine dip for protein & glucose + send for C&S**
5. **CBC**

Should all pregnant patients be screened for trichomonas?

No –
Not unless there are symptoms

If a patient is on suppressive therapy for herpes, is transmission of HSV still possible?

Yes

(Recent studies show dramatic reductions in transmission with suppression, though, and experts disagree as to whether asymptomatic transmission in a vigilant patient is really possible or not)

Which adolescent women are at increased risk for (later) cervical cancer? (2)	1. Multiple partners 2. STD history
Can Pap smears be used to screen for STDs?	No! – It only screens for cervical cancer
Should Pap smears be done while the woman is menstruating?	Preferably not – It can make cytology interpretation more difficult
Is it all right to collect a Pap smear when evaluating for a possible STD?	Yes – Although they often need to be repeated due to inflammatory changes
If it may be difficult to interpret, should you collect a Pap smear when evaluating for a possible STD?	Yes – As long as it would ordinarily have been time for one
When must an abnormal Pap smear be followed up with colposcopy/biopsy?	ASC-H (Atypical squamous cells cannot exclude high-grade changes) HSIL (high-grade squamous intraepithelial lesions) AGC (Atypical glandular cells)
Which abnormal Pap smears can be followed up with a repeat Pap smear at 12 & 24 months, and not investigated further if the repeats are all right?	ASC-US finding
In what situation could an abnormal Pap smear NOT be followed up with further smears or colposcopy?	If HPV testing is done & the result is negative (you may then resume routine testing in women <24 years old)
When doing a pelvic exam, when should the Pap smear be collected?	Last (Unlike cultures, other parts of the exam won't affect it)
If an adolescent female has mucopurulent discharge at the cervix, can a Pap smear still be performed?	Yes

In adults, yearly Pap smears are not always recommended. What about for sexually active adolescents?	No routine Pap smears are recommended until the patient reaches age 21 years
	(Note: This is a change! Previous yearly Pap smears were recommended for sexually active adolescents)
If a young person has a myocardial infarction, what abuse issue should you always consider?	Cocaine
What growth problem can anabolic steroids cause for the skeleton?	Short stature – Due to premature closure of the epiphyses
Which organ is at increased risk for cancer after anabolic steroid use?	The liver (hepatocellular carcinoma)
Which organ is at risk for acute inflammation with anabolic steroid use?	The liver (hepatitis)
What clues on physical exam suggest anabolic steroid use? (1 general finding, and 3 skin findings)	• General – weight gain (due to both increased mass & fluid retention) • Skin – acne, hirsutism, & striae
For males, what reproductive organ changes suggest possible anabolic steroid use? (3)	1. Gynecomastia 2. Testicular atrophy 3. Azoospermia
What psychiatric impact can anabolic steroids have on adolescents? (4)	1. Depression 2. Mania 3. Rage 4. Change in libido
If an adolescent presents with odynophagia & "heartburn" that is bad enough he has difficulty sleeping, what should you always ask about? **(popular boards topic)**	**Acne medications**

Why would acne medication lead to odynophagia & heartburn?	**Tetracyclines are famous for causing esophageal irritation is the pill lodges there** **(aka "pill esophagitis")**
How are patients supposed to prevent tetracyclines from lodging in their esophagus?	**Drink a full (8 or 12 ounce) glass of water with the pill**
If your adolescent patient is having so much discomfort that s/he can't sleep, due to a tetracycline pill that irritated the esophagus, what should you do?	**Pain control as best you can – It will resolve in time**
Will antacid medications help with the pain of pill esophagitis?	**No** **(The pain is not due to reflux)**
In addition to taking tetracyclines with lots of water, what else should you tell patients to try to prevent pill esophagitis?	**Don't take the pill at bedtime (Gravity will help it to move into the stomach, if your patient is up and about)**
What are the three most commonly tested antibiotics that you generally *should not give to pregnant patients?*	1. **Erythromycin *estolate* (liver toxicity issues in mother – other erythromycin forms are alright)** 2. **Tetracyclines (fetal tooth discoloration)** 3. **Fluoroquinolones including ciprofloxacin (cartilage/bone issues)**
Are there any important cognitive effects with marijuana use?	↓ **short-term memory** ↓ **driving performance (impaired coordination)** ↓ **judgment (difficulty thinking and problem solving)** **Time & distance perception is distorted**

What endocrine effects are associated with marijuana use?	↓ **testosterone** **(& ↓ spermatogenesis)**
	↓ **growth hormone**
	possible ↓ thyroid function (likely transient)
Bleeding & pain 5–8 weeks after menses suggests what possible diagnosis?	**Ectopic pregnancy** (The previous menses were probably abnormal, & the interval is right for an ectopic to get big enough to become symptomatic)
How is ectopic pregnancy treated? (2)	1. Surgically 2. Methotrexate & serial HCGs (quantitative) *if very early & non-ruptured*
What is the most conservative way to manage an ectopic pregnancy, and usually the preferred way on the boards?	Surgery
When ectopic pregnancy is suspected or confirmed, what management is needed while the patient waits for the OR?	Treat the patient like a trauma patient – 2 large-bore IV lines & give crystalloid (NS or lactated ringers)
Is vaginal bleeding associated with ectopic pregnancy?	Yes
If a gestational sac can be seen on ultrasound (US), does that confirm an intrauterine pregnancy?	No – You must see fetal/embryonic parts
What is the minimum finding the ultrasonographer must see to document an intrauterine pregnancy?	Yolk sac
At how many weeks can a gestational sac usually be seen on US?	• 6 weeks transabdominal • 4.5 weeks transvaginal ultrasound
What US findings confirm an IUP (intrauterine pregnancy)?	• Yolk sac • Fetal pole • Fetal heart

Where do 90 % of ectopic pregnancies implant?

Distal ampulla of the fallopian tube

What mechanical contraceptive is notorious for increasing the risk of ectopic pregnancy?

IUDs
(intrauterine devices)

A past history of what two medical problems means the patient is at increased risk of ectopic pregnancy?

Pelvic inflammatory disease

Or

Prior ectopic pregnancy

A history of what general type of surgery put the patient at increased risk for ectopic pregnancy?

Pelvic surgery

(& especially fallopian tube surgery)

What is a "missed" abortion?

1. Pregnant female
2. Fetal death <20 weeks
3. All products retained (no bleeding)

What is the treatment for a missed abortion?
(abbreviated on charts as "missed ab")

D & C
(dilation & curettage)

What are the two most concerning complications of missed abortions?

Sepsis

&

Disseminated intravascular coagulation (DIC)

What types of microbes are present in septic abortion?

Polymicrobial –
Including anaerobes

How do you define a "threatened" abortion?
   (4 components)

1. Pregnant female
2. Vaginal bleeding
3. *Closed os*
4. <20 weeks' gestation

If a patient presents with a threatened abortion, what treatment & diagnostic procedures are required?

Treatment – bed rest/pelvic rest

Diagnostic – check blood type
(Rh Ig may be needed)

(Note: Ultrasound of fetus is not generally indicated, but is often done anyway)

What is an "incomplete" abortion?

What it sounds like –
Pregnant female with vaginal bleeding & tissue at os

Or

Some products of conception/vaginal lining are still in the uterus, but the pregnancy is no longer viable

What is the treatment for an incomplete abortion?

D & C
(dilation & curettage)

One final category. What is an "inevitable" abortion?

1. Pregnant female
2. Bleeding
3. Membrane ruptured
4. os *open*
5. <20 weeks

If your patient is diagnosed with an "inevitable" abortion, what are the possible outcomes for that situation?
(2)

1. Completed spontaneous abortion
2. Incomplete abortion (requiring D & C)

If bleeding is unusually heavy or prolonged in an inevitable abortion, what will most practitioners choose to do?

D & C

A pregnant female had some pain & bleeding, passed clots & tissue, and now has less pain & bleeding. What is her diagnosis?

Completed abortion
(no treatment required)

If a woman has a miscarriage in the first trimester, and she doesn't have excessive bleeding, should you still check her blood type? Why or why not?

**Yes –
If she is Rh–, she will need a small standard dose of RhoGam**

What test is used to determine the dose of Rhogam needed in Rh– women >12 weeks pregnant after miscarriage or trauma?

Kleihauer-Betke

What is the Kleihauer-Betke test looking for?	Fetal RBCs in the maternal circulation
Bed rest & pelvic rest would be appropriate instructions for what abortion type?	Threatened abortion (Note: It is not clear whether this is helpful or not, but it is generally recommended)
If an Rh− mother has already been sensitized to Rh+ blood, how should you assess the well-being of the fetus during pregnancy? (4)	1. Determine the father's Rh status 2. Check maternal antibody titers – high or rising titer means trouble 3. Perform serial amniocenteses to check the bilirubin level OR check the middle cerebral artery peak systolic velocities to noninvasively estimate the level of anemia 4. Transfuse as needed (via umbilicus)
When can minigam (miniRhogam) be used?	Rh− Moms 12 weeks pregnant or less
At how many gestational weeks does the uterus emerge from the pelvis?	End of the 12th week
If the uterine fundus is at the umbilicus, how many gestational weeks should the pregnancy be?	20 weeks
When a pregnancy is at 20 weeks gestation, how many centimeters should it be from the public symphysis to the umbilicus?	20 cm
In the first 2 months of pregnancy, how rapidly should HCG levels rise?	Doubles every 2 days
How rapidly the HCG level fall after either abortion or delivery?	Drops by half every 2 days (after delivery can last 3 weeks)
How soon after ovulation is HCG detectable, if a pregnancy occurs?	About 8 days after ovulation

What constitutes a "positive culdocentesis?"

Non-clotting blood
(with a hematocrit >15 %)

Found in the "pouch of Douglas" just behind the uterus

Are culdocenteses commonly performed?

No –
But it is still tested

What would culdocenteses mainly be used for?

Mainly looking for bleeding near the uterus –
such as from a ruptured ectopic pregnancy

(occasionally to evaluate for PID)

How is pyelonephritis managed during pregnancy?
(3)

1. Admit
2. IV antibiotics
   (usually ampicillin & gentamicin)
3. D/C on PO Abx after afebrile 48 h
   (treat for 14 days total)

Outpatient therapy is still NOT recommended for pregnant patients, except in very specific circumstances

Although contraceptive sponges are not commonly used anymore, if a question should appear about them, what significant risks are there for women using the sponge?

1. Dislodgement –
   especially for parous
   women
2. Toxic shock syndrome
   (if left in place too
   long)

How effective are spermicides when used by themselves?

About 75 % (per year of use)

What concern about the use of spermicides has developed for patients, especially is the patient is exposed to more than one partner?

Small increased risk of acquiring STDs due to irritation of mucosal surfaces
(Also does not prevent transmission of STDs)

Nonoxynol-9, the most common spermicide, should not be used in which situations?

Partner with HIV (increases risk of transmission)

More than one time per day (due to mucosal irritation)

For anal sex (irritation & breakdown of mucosal barriers)

Patients who have multiple partners (increased risk of STD acquisition due to mucosal irritation & breakdown)

A pruritic (itchy) vulvar area that does not respond to antifungal creams should be evaluated for what?
(3)

1. Vulvar intraepithelial neoplasia (VIN)
2. Melanoma
3. Paget's disease (of the skin – usually seen in adults)

How is vulvar intraepithelial neoplasia different in younger vs. older women?

It is usually multifocal & very aggressive in younger women

(Single focus & generally unaggressive in older women)

Are vulvar intraepithelial neoplasia & Paget's disease the same thing?

No –
VIN is associated with
HPV . . .

Paget's disease is inflammatory (but still premalignant)

Explain the staging system for cervical cancer

0 – in situ only
1 – cervix only
2 – involves adjacent areas but *not* the pelvic wall or lower 1/3 of vagina
3 – pelvic wall, lower 1/3 of vagina, or kidney affected
4 – outside the pelvis, or involving the rectal or bladder mucosa

It is most important to know stages 0, 1, & 2

The majority of malignant ovarian tumors are what type?	Serous Mnemonic: Serious (!) tumors
Are the majority of ovarian tumors malignant or benign?	Most are benign
What is "stage 0" cervical cancer?	Carcinoma in situ
Strawberry cervix & gray-yellow "frothy" discharge = ?	Trichomonas
Fishy odor & "clue cells" = what diagnosis?	Bacterial vaginosis (aka Gardnerella)
How do you treat trichomonas? (2)	Metronidazole Or Tinidazole
If a patient has trichomonas, should his or her partner also be treated?	Yes
Should you treat bacterial vaginosis?	Yes – Metronidazole Or Clindamycin
Should partners of bacterial vaginosis partners be treated?	Only if balanitis is present – It is not always acquired as an STD *(Balanitis is local inflammation at the glans)*
Can metronidazole be used for pregnant women?	No – Not on the boards (actually depends on the trimester, but better not to)
What is a corpus luteal cyst?	A cyst that develops in the last 2 weeks of the menstrual cycle (in the area that ovulated)

How should a corpus luteal cyst be treated?	Symptomatic only, if needed (in rare instances, surgery may be needed to control bleeding, but most cases are managed conservatively & outpatient)
What is the main risk factor for ovarian torsion?	Cyst on the ovary (usually 3 cm or larger)
What are the main problems associated with ovarian cysts? (4)	1. Abdominal pain 2. Cyst rupture (painful, but not dangerous) 3. Torsion (threatens fertility) 4. Hemorrhage (sometimes dangerous)
Is vaginal bleeding associated with ovarian torsion?	No – Not usually
What is the most common site for endometriosis?	The ovary
Constant pelvic pain associated with menses suggests what diagnosis?	Endometriosis
What is the most common cause of dysfunctional uterine bleeding (DUB)?	Anovulatory cycle
What molecule will be found in the amniotic fluid if surfactant is being made?	Phosphatidylglycerol
What ratio is used to determine whether fetal lungs are mature?	The L:S Or Lecithin to sphingomyelin ratio
How high should the lung maturity ratio be, to ensure that fetal lungs are ready for delivery?	≥ 2.0
What factors promote fetal surfactant production, in general terms?	Things that stress the fetus

What maternal endocrine disorder accelerates fetal surfactant production?	Hyperthyroidism
What three things that start with "p" stress the fetus, leading to early surfactant production?	Premature rupture of membranes (prolonged) Preeclampsia Placental insufficiency
Giving the mother which medication encourages early surfactant production?	Steroids
Moms addicted to which class of drugs tend to have early babies with early surfactant production?	Narcotics (Drug addiction stresses fetuses!)
Which airway medication is associated with early surfactant production by the fetus?	Theophylline Mnemonic: Assume that it's stressful for a fetus if Mom has reactive airway disease requiring theophylline!
What factors delay fetal surfactant production? (2)	1. Hyperglycemia 2. Hyperinsulinemia
If a pregnant woman presents for prenatal care and is *not* rubella immune, should she be immunized at that time?	No – The vaccine carries a risk of active infection (very small risk, though)
What does "overflow incontinence" refer to?	Inadequate bladder contractions cause retention of urine, and intermittent incontinence with overdistention
What does "urge incontinence" refer to?	The bladder muscle sometimes contracts "on its own" Buzzword: "Detrusor instability!"
What does "stress incontinence" refer to?	Incontinence during Valsalva (misalignment of structures renders the muscular floor of the bladder less effective)

What is the "puerperium?"

The 6 weeks following delivery

What is the main component of Kallman's syndrome?

Congenital absence of GnRH

What unusual physical finding is associated with Kallman's syndrome?

Anosmia – or severely decreased sense of smell

(This can also happen due to tumor or trauma, but then it is not officially "Kallman's syndrome.")

A snowstorm appearance on a pregnancy ultrasound indicates what diagnosis?

Molar pregnancy

What *is* a molar pregnancy?

The chorionic villi grow, but there is no fetus

A pregnant woman with exaggerated symptoms of pregnancy, and first or second trimester bleeding may have what diagnosis?

Molar pregnancy!

What significant complications are molar pregnancy patients at increased risk to develop?

Choriocarcinoma

&

Preeclampsia

Preeclampsia or eclampsia in the first half of pregnancy usually indicates what underlying problem?

Molar pregnancy

(eclampsia = seizures)
(preeclampsia = protein in urine, edema, hypertension, risk for seizures)

If a patient presents complaining of passing "grape-like" clusters per vagina, you should think of what diagnosis?

Molar pregnancy

The buzzword for the gross appearance of a molar pregnancy is _____?

Grape-like clusters

How should a molar pregnancy be treated?
(2 items)

1. D & C (dilation & curettage, to clean out uterine contents)
2. Metastatic evaluation (for occult choriocarcinoma)

Painful vaginal bleeding in a late trimester pregnant female suggests what diagnosis?

Abruptio placenta

In a suspected placental abruption, how reassuring is a negative ultrasound?

Not very

(abruptions are often in the fundus or posterior areas, and are hard to see on US)

What drug of abuse may cause placental abruption?

Cocaine

What routine evaluation must you _avoid_ in a vaginally bleeding third trimester pregnant woman?

Pelvic exam! –
You could stick your fingers into the placenta & cause very tough to control bleeding!

Pain*less* vaginal bleeding late in pregnancy may indicate what worrisome problem?

Placenta previa

Why shouldn't you do a pelvic exam on someone who has a placenta previa?

Your fingers could tear the placenta – producing much more bleeding

What if the patient has abruption? Will doing a pelvic exam worsen that bleeding?

Generally not –
We don't do it because we can't be sure that it's not a previa

If a third-trimester pregnant woman has dark red vaginal bleeding, which is more likely, previa or abruption?

Abruption
(The blood takes time to work its way out, so it's darker)

In placental abruption, will the patient always have vaginal bleeding?

No –
Sometimes the blood is contained within the uterus

How is abruption managed?

Depends on the size and gestational age –

If possible, bed rest & observation
If the abruption is too large, delivery

What related condition may require management in an abruption patient?

Hypertension
(may cause abruption, or worsen abruption)

The bleeding of placenta previa is usually described as _____ and _____.

Painless

&

Bright red

How is placenta previa treated, if there isn't any vaginal bleeding?

1. **Observation** (some placentas politely move to a better location over time)
2. **C-section delivery, if previa is still present at term**

How is placenta previa treated if there is active bleeding?

Bedrest

&

Tocolytics to delay delivery

Can a placenta previa patient be allowed to attempt a vaginal delivery?

No –
Delivering *through* the placenta is not workable!!

What is the most common surgical emergency of pregnancy?

Appendicitis!

Why is appendicitis harder than usual to diagnose in pregnant patients?

Mainly because the appendix is often not in the usual location in advanced pregnancy

Where will appendicitis often cause abdominal pain in pregnancy?

Right upper quadrant –
Because the appendix is actually displaced to the right upper quadrant in later pregnancy

In general, is the pregnant patient's blood pressure low, normal, or elevated?

Low to normal

If a pregnant woman has a blood pressure of 140/90, should you be concerned (assuming she has no previous history of hypertension)?

Yes –
This is significantly high for a pregnant woman

What is the HELLP syndrome?

Hemolytic anemia
Elevated Liver enzymes
Low Platelets
(in pregnant women, of course)

Will the coagulation test be abnormal in HELLP patients?

No

Most pregnant women have some edema. What makes the edema of preeclampsia different?

It affects non-dependent areas also (hands, face, etc.)

Which patients are most likely to develop preeclampsia?
  (5 factors)

1. Primigravida
2. Very young or very old mothers
3. >20 weeks' gestation
4. Multiple gestations
5. Diabetics

How is eclampsia different from preeclampsia?

Seizures happen!!!

What is the treatment for eclampsia/ severe pre-eclampsia?

Delivery

(Mild preeclampsia at <37 weeks – expectant management due to comorbidities related to prematurity)

If an eclamptic woman is unstable (acutely), should you perform a C-section to deliver her?

No –
Stabilize first

How are seizures treated in an eclamptic patient?

Magnesium
(2–4 g over 20 min)

What is the most typical agent used to control blood pressure in pregnant, hypertensive patients?

Hydralazine –
(labetolol & nifedipine are also fine)

If too much magnesium is given to a pregnant patient, what complications may occur?

Respiratory arrest

(+ poor reflexes & floppy muscles overall)

What is the most common, preventable, cause of perinatal mortality?

Pregnancy-induced hypertension *(sometimes abbreviated PIH)*

If a pregnant patient has asymptomatic pyuria, or bacteriuria, should you treat it?

Yes –
10-day course

(No treatment needed in a nonpregnant patient)

Which typical UTI medications must you avoid in pregnancy?

Quinolones

&

Sulfa (third trimester only)

Why are possible UTIs treated so aggressively in pregnant patients?

High risk of pyelonephritis

Is it alright to give tetanus vaccinations to pregnant patients?

Yes

(only live virus vaccines are a problem – this one is not live)

The guiding concept in treating a pregnant trauma patient is . . .?

Stabilize the mother to help the baby

If a pregnant patient is hypotensive & lying down, what should you try *first*, to improve BP?

Left lateral decubitus position
(moves pressure away from the IVC → better venous return)

Labor before what week of pregnancy is definitely considered "preterm?"

36 weeks

How is preterm labor typically treated?

Bedrest

&

Tocolytics
(e.g., magnesium sulfate, nifedipine, or indomethacin if earlier than 32 weeks)

Which test allows you to know how much RhoGam is needed for Rh– mothers who may have been exposed to Rh+ blood?

Kleihauer-Betke

Will patients with mastitis have a fever?

Usually, yes

How is mastitis treated?	Warm compresses, NSAIDS & Antibiotics
If a postpartum or post-abortion patient develops a fever, abdominal pain, & foul-smelling discharge, what is the likely diagnosis?	Endometritis
How is endometritis usually treated? (3 steps)	1. Admit 2. Broad-spectrum antibiotics (usually a polymicrobial infection) 3. D & C if retained products are suspected
What vitamin supplement should all women of reproductive age take & why?	• **Folate** • **To prevent neural tube defects**
Which virus must you be sure a pregnant woman has immunity to?	**Rubella –** **Do an antibody screen**
What are the five parts of the biophysical profile of the fetus?	1. Nonstress test (heart rate variability observation) 2. Fetal breathing movement 3. Fetal body movement 4. Amniotic fluid index 5. Fetal muscle tone
How often should you get a biophysical profile in the third trimester of a high-risk pregnancy?	Twice per week
If the biophysical profile gives concerning results, what is the next step in management?	A "contraction stress test" (fetal heart rate is monitored while oxytocin is given to cause uterine contraction)
How is a bad result on the contraction stress test defined?	Late decelerations with contractions

What is the next step in management if late decelerations with little variability are observed with contractions in a contraction stress test?

C-section delivery

What are the main *consequences* of oligohydramnios?
(3)

1. Pulmonary hypoplasia
2. Skin & skeletal problems (due to compression)
3. Hypoxia (due to umbilical cord compression)

What are the main maternal consequences of polyhydramnios?
(2)

Maternal dyspnea
(not enough space to breathe)

&

Uterine atony
(overstretched uterus)

Post-term fetuses may develop which abnormality in regard to the amount of amniotic fluid present?

Oligohydramnios

IUGR (intrauterine growth retardation) fetuses are prone to which amniotic fluid abnormality?

Oligohydramnios

Neural tube defect fetuses, those with GI abnormalities, and multiple gestations, are prone to what amniotic fluid abnormality?

Polyhydramnios

How do you recognize an "early deceleration" on a fetal monitor strip?

Fetal heart deceleration & uterine contraction peak at the same time

What does an early deceleration usually indicate?

**Normal vagal response to head compression
(with descent into the vagina/cervix)**

Which type of deceleration is most worrisome, and what does it indicate?

- Late
- Uteroplacental insufficiency (not enough circulation to fetus)

A fetal scalp pH of less than what number is reason for rapid C-section delivery?

7.2

What type of deceleration is most common?	Variable (meaning that decelerations have no stable relationship to contractions)
What do variable decelerations indicate?	Umbilical cord compression
How might epidural anesthesia contribute to late decelerations?	Epidural sometimes drop the mother's blood pressure, increasing the likelihood of uteroplacental insufficiency
If late or variable decelerations occur during labor, how should they be managed? (4 steps)	1. Left lateral decubitus position 2. O_2 3. Stop oxytocin (if it's on) 4. IV fluids
What is the half-life of oxytocin?	About 5 min
If initial strategies to improve abnormal fetal heart rate or decelerations are not successful, what is the next step in management?	Check fetal scalp pH
What is a normal heart rate for a term fetus/infant?	110–160 with good variability
What is the second stage of labor?	Full dilation to birth of baby (pushing phase)
The first stage of labor is the only one with two parts. What are they?	Latent (0–3 cm) Active (3–10 cm, full dilation)
What is "arrested labor?"	No cervical change over a 2-h period (Does not mean your patient is handcuffed!)
If no reason is found for arrest of labor, what are the next steps in management? (3 options)	1. Give oxytocin 2. Use prostaglandin gel 3. Perform amniotomy
What endocrine disorder can oxytocin sometimes mimic?	SIADH (hyponatremia) *Oxytocin has an ADH-type effect*

Which antibody type crosses the placenta?	Only IgG (Usually IgM is given as a distractor – remember that IgM looks like a giant snowflake or a whole bunch of "Ms" placed in a circle. It's much too large to cross.)
How is hyperemesis gravidarum treated?	1. Small, frequent meals 2. IV fluid & antiemetics PRN 3. Decrease social stressors, if possible
Rh incompatibility may lead to what fetal disorder?	Hydrops fetalis (edema, ascites, & anemia)
Trauma to a breast, followed by a local mass, is probably the result of what process?	Fat necrosis – will resolve in time
Should you suspect cancer if a patient presents with bilateral nipple discharge?	No
Nipple discharge due to carcinoma typically has what two characteristics?	Unilateral & Bloody
What is the main endocrine abnormality in polycystic ovary syndrome?	High androgens (Usually hairy females with irregular menses)
How is premenstrual syndrome (PMS) treated in adolescents?	**NSAIDs, diuretics for symptomatic relief, and occasionally antidepressants or antianxiety medications** **(OCPs are sometimes used, but studies to date have not shown them to be effective)**
What are the two most common causes of dysfunctional uterine bleeding in adolescents?	**Anovulatory cycle** **&** **Polycystic ovaries**

How can heavy dysfunctional uterine bleeding (DUB) be treated? (2 options)	1. Estrogen 2. D & C
How is mild DUB treated? (2 options)	1. Oral contraceptives 2. Progesterone or estrogen supplementation alone
In terms of age, how is primary amenorrhea defined?	No menses by age 16 years
How rapidly should menarche follow development of secondary sexual characteristics?	**Within 2 years**
If breast development has occurred, but not menses or axillary/pubic hair development, what disorder should you consider?	Androgen insensitivity (genetically XY)
If a patient complains of either primary or secondary amenorrhea, and is not pregnant, what should you do to evaluate the situation?	Give progesterone – Bleeding should follow withdrawal if the uterus & estrogen status are normal
What is adenomyosis?	Endometrial glands in the uterine muscle
How does adenomyosis cause problems?	Pain & increased bleeding with menses
How is adenomyosis treated?	GnRH agonists Or Hysterectomy (if symptoms very severe)

Index

Printed in the United States
By Bookmasters